Foot &
Ankle
Pearls

Foot & Ankle Pearls

RICHARD M. JAY, D.P.M., FACFAS
Professor of Foot and Ankle Orthopedics
Temple University—School of Podiatric Medicine
Director of Foot and Ankle Surgical Residency Program
  and Medical Education
Graduate Hospital
Philadelphia, Pennsylvania

HANLEY & BELFUS, INC. / Philadelphia

Publisher: HANLEY & BELFUS, INC.
               Medical Publishers
               210 S. 13th Street
               Philadelphia, PA 19107
               (215) 546-7293, 800-962-1892
               FAX (215) 790-9330
               Website: http://www.hanleyandbelfus.com

Library of Congress Cataloging-in-Publication Data

Foot and ankle pearls / edited by Richard M. Jay.
        p. ; cm.—(The pearls series)
     Includes bibliographical references and index.
     ISBN 1-56053-445-1 (alk. paper)
     1. Foot—Diseases—Case studies. 2. Ankle—Diseases—Case studies. I. Jay, Richard M.
II. Series
     [DNLM: 1. Foot Diseases—diagnosis—Case Report. 2. Foot Diseases—diagnosis—Problems
and Exercises. 3. Ankle Injuries—diagnosis—Case Report. 4. Ankle Injuries—diagnosis—Problems
and Exercises. 5. Foot Injuries—diagnosis—Case Report. 6. Foot Injuries—diagnosis—Problems
and Exercises. WE 18.2 F687 2001]
     RC951 .F66 2002
     617.5'85—dc21
                                                                              2001039937

Printed in Canada

FOOT & ANKLE PEARLS   ISBN 1-56053-445-1

Last digit is the print number: 9 8 7 6 5 4 3 2 1

CONTENTS

CONTRIBUTORS

Richard M. Jay, D.P.M., FACFAS
Professor of Foot and Ankle Orthopedics, Temple University–School of Podiatric Medicine, Philadelphia; Director of Foot and Ankle Surgical Residency Program and Medical Education, Graduate Hospital, Philadelphia, Pennsylvania

The Graduate Hospital Foot and Ankle Residency Program
Philadelphia, Pennsylvania
Jeffrey DeLott, D.P.M.
Shane Hollawell, D.P.M.
Robert McConekey, D.P.M.
Michael Rayno, D.P.M.
Brian Rell, D.P.M.
Thomas Landino, D.P.M.
Dawn Pfieffer, D.P.M.
Barry White, D.P.M.
Jodi Schoenhaus, D.P.M.

PREFACE

Foot and Ankle Pearls is the latest volume in the highly popular Pearls Series®. This book is a compilation of interesting and challenging cases seen at the Graduate Hospital in Philadelphia, and it provides valuable information not readily available in standard textbooks. Each case is unique and illustrates one or more diagnostic or therapeutic issues confronting the clinician. It is also "interactive" in that the reader, based on the information represented (usually relating to a pain syndrome), is asked to make a diagnosis. The diagnosis is later revealed and discussed, and aspects that are especially important are captured and listed at the end of each case as "Clinical Pearls."

I have availed myself of the expertise of the Graduate Hospital Foot and Ankle surgical residents, as they have a keen and observant eye for interesting cases and are among the brightest and most energetic physicians I know. It was natural to ask them for help in putting together this book. Thanks to Hanley & Belfus for allowing me to reprint a few cases from *Rheumatology Pearls* and *Infectious Disease Pearls*.

Enjoy!

Richard M. Jay, DPM, FACFAS
EDITOR

PATIENT 1

A 43-year-old woman with a painful and swollen great toe

The patient presents with a 3-day history of pain and swelling in the left big toe joint. She says, "It hurts to even have the sheets touch my toe." The patient denies any history of trauma to the left foot and states that she saw her primary doctor, who started her on indomethacin 50mg BID. When relief had not been obtained 2 days later, she came to the emergency department for treatment. The patient is without a significant past medical history.

Physical Examination: Vital signs: normal. General: mild distress. HEENT: normal. Cardiac: regular rate, no murmurs. Chest: clear breath sounds. Abdomen: soft, nontender. Extremities: palpable pedal pulses bilaterally; a swollen, reddened, tender left 1st MTP joint of the left foot, with 1+ non-pitting edema. Neurologic: intact.

Laboratory Findings: CBC with differential: WBC 13,300/µl (4000–10,000 normal); lymphocytes 5000/µl (1000–4500 normal). Radiograph of left foot (see figure): erosion of the first metatarsal head with sclerotic bone exhibiting a martel sign. Serum urinalysis: normal. ESR 45 mm/hr (increased). Arthrocentesis of left 1st MTP joint: increased WBC, specifically neutrophils 85 (0–24 normal); monosodium urate crystals (needle-shaped and display a negative birefringence under polarizing light microscopy).

Question: What syndrome explains this patient's signs and symptoms?

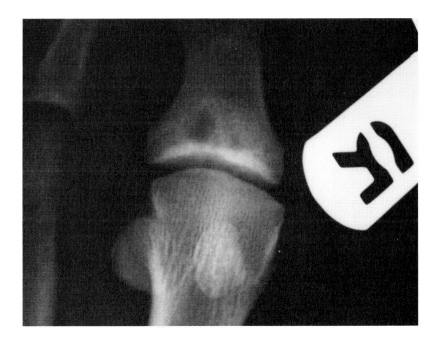

Diagnosis: Acute gouty arthritis

Discussion: Gout is a disorder of purine metabolism characterized by hyperuricemia and the deposition of monosodium urate crystals in joints. Attacks may be precipitated by trauma, surgery, fasting, infection, and medications such as diuretics. Gout is usually monoarticular and predominately affects the joints of the lower extremity, specifically the 1st MTP joint. This disease is widely dispersed among many races and has a higher incidence in men vs. women typically over the age of 30. Women who are affected are usually postmenopausal. The discrepancy between the sexes is believed to be due to the action that estrogen plays in promoting renal excretion of uric acid.

Pathogenesis involves uric acid, either from ingestion of foods containing purines (e.g., shellfish, beef, alcoholic beverages) or endogenous synthesis of purine nucleotides. Humans lack the enzyme uricase, which oxidizes uric acid to allantoin. Under steady-state conditions, renal excretion is the major route of uric acid disposal (approximately two-thirds), and bacterial oxidization of urate into the gut accounts for the remaining one-third. Two factors—either alone or in combination—contribute substantially to the hyperuricemia of gout: Increased uric acid production due to an abnormality in the metabolism (HGPRT deficiency), and diminished uric acid secretion by the kidney.

The pathology of acute gout arthritis involves urate crystallizing as a monosodium salt and oversaturating joint tissue. Sodium urate becomes less soluble at lower temperatures, which may explain why the urate crystals predispose to deposition in areas such as the toe joints and earlobes. The urate crystals initiate and sustain intense attacks of acute inflammation because of their ability to stimulate the release of several inflammatory mediators.

Signs and symptoms include redness, heat, swelling, and tenderness of the affected joint, often with prodromal irritability and a sudden onset of pain in the early hours of the morning. The patient typically remarks that it hurts to even have the sheets of the bed touch the area. Serum uric acid levels may or may not be elevated, and often there is an increased serum WBC as well as an elevated ESR acutely. Radiographic findings are usually normal at this stage, but may demonstrate soft tissue swelling and joint effusions. Definitive diagnosis is established by arthrocentesis of the joint and synovial fluid analysis. The presence of monosodium urate crystals that are needle-shaped and display negative birefringence under polarizing light microscopy is definitive. Also, synovial fluid leukocytes are elevated, with a predomination of neutrophils.

Treatment consists of the oral administration of NSAIDs, such as indomethacin, up to 75mg sustained-release BID and/or colchicine. Colchicine is a very toxic drug with GI effects such as nausea, vomiting, diarrhea, and cramping when administered orally. It has been suggested that a prompt response to colchicine is diagnostic of gout. However, note that other arthropathies also respond to colchicine. Also, if it is started 24 hours after onset of an attack, the response can be variable. Other treatment options include an intra-articular injection of cortiosteroids, administration of ACTH, rest, and elevation of affected area.

In the present patient, a treatment course of colchicine provided a marked reduction of pain after 5 hours.

Clinical Pearls

1. In acute gouty arthritis, ESR and serum WBCs are often elevated.
2. Presence of needle-shaped monosodium urate crystals with negative birefringence in synovial aspirate is diagnostic.
3. Acute gouty arthritis usually is monoarticular and is preceded by prodromal irritability.
4. It affects more males than females over the age of 30.

REFERENCES
1. Isselbacher KJ, Braunwald E, Wilson JD, et al (eds): Harrison's Principles of Internal Medicine, 14th ed. New York, Mc-Graw-Hill, 1998.
2. Klippel JH, Weyand CM, Wortmann RL (eds): Primer on the Rheumatic Diseases, 11th ed. Atlanta, GA, Arthritis Foundation, 1997.

PATIENT 2

A 43-year-old man with constant heel pain

A 43-year-old man presents with a 2- to 3-month history of constant left plantar and lateral heel pain. He relates that he has experienced intermittent foot and bilateral knee pain for several years. Surgical arthroscopy was performed on his bilateral knees, with mild to moderate pain relief. However, pain in the left heel has persisted with both ambulation and nonweight-bearing, and has become mildly progressive.

Physical Examination: Temperature 98.6° F; pulse 78; respirations 16; blood pressure 150/80. HEENT: normal. Lungs: clear. Cardiac: regular. Abdomen: nontender. Skin: normal, with healed arthroscopy portals on the left and right knees. Musculoskeletal: pain on palpation of plantar medial and lateral tubercles of left calcaneus, and on lateral compression of left calcaneus; nontender plantar fascia; manual muscle testing of lower extremity normal.

Laboratory Findings: CBC with differential: normal. Chemistry profile: normal. Lung function tests: normal. PT/PTT: normal. Cholesterol: 209 (120–199 normal). *Pathology:* Gross specimen—2.5 × 1.5 × 1 cm aggregate of yellow bony tissue. Microscopic specimen—cystic lesion with dense, hyalinized wall containing area of bony sclerosis, some hemosiderin pigment deposition, and areas of increased vascularity; surrounding bone showed fatty replacement of marrow. *Imaging:* Radiographs of right foot—no osseous pathology; left foot (see left figure)—large intra-calcaneal bone cyst of the body, with well-circumscribed borders. MRI of left foot (see right figure)—interosseous significantly lobulated calcaneal bone cyst with marked increase in signal intensity, indicative of high fluid content on T2-weighted image; signal intensity comparable to subcutaneous fat and adjacent intramedullary bone on proton density–weighted image.

Question: What is the most likely cause of the patient's heel pain?

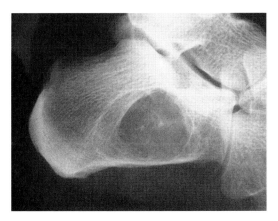 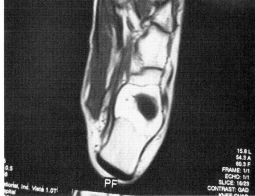

Diagnosis: Intraosseous lipoma of the calcaneus

Discussion: Intraosseous lipomas of the calcaneus are extremely rare. They are more commonly found in the lower extremity than the upper extremity. The bones most often affected are the metaphyseal regions of long bones such as the femur, tibia, and fibula. Irregular bones such as the spine and calcaneus, however, can be affected. The percentage of all bone tumors occurring in the foot is less than 2%. The majority of intraosseous lipomas of the calcaneus are typically found within the central portion or body. Though uncommon, the diagnosis of calcaneal bone cyst should be considered in the differential diagnosis of atypical heel pain.

The diagnosis of calcaneal bone cyst is based on the patient's history, clinical findings, physical exam, and radiologic evaluation. There are many different etiologies of heel pain. Note that the accurate diagnosis of itraosseous lipoma can lead to a proper and effective treatment for the patient.

The present patient was taken to the operating room, and an excisional biopsy was performed through a curved lateral incision over the calcaneus. A lateral cortical window was created over the underlying cystic lesion with a sagittal saw. The lipomatous lobular mass was removed en toto and sent to pathology for frozen specimen determination and subsequent histological evaluation. The sclerotic wall of the cyst was aggressively curetted. The void was filled with "ground down" mixture of autogenic iliac bone graft and allogenic corticocancellous bone graft chips because of the large size of the intraosseous deficit. The cortical window was replaced and secured with an orthosorb pin. Closure was then performed in sequential fashion.

The patient was immobilized for approximately 6 weeks in a cast, and then given a cam walker. Progressive weight-bearing began at approximately 8 weeks, and at the 3-month follow-up the patient was almost 100% pain-free in his left foot. He returned to full activity without limitations, only occasionally experiencing discomfort in his left knee and foot if swelling occurred.

Clinical Pearls

1. There are several hypotheses, but the true etiology of an intraosseous lipoma is unknown.

2. The pain of intraosseous lipomas can vary from intermittent to constant, dull aching. Upon palpation there may be tenderness in the involved bone, and symptoms may last for years.

3. MRI and CT scan can be extremely helpful in outlining the borders of the lesion and determining the extent of intraosseous involvement. They can also be very useful when planning the surgical excision of the lesion.

4. There is a risk for pathological fracture of the calcaneus when a large tumor or intraosseous cyst is present. Therefore excisional biopsy with curettage and bone grafting is often recommended.

5. Though the lesion is benign, the possibility of malignancy exists, either as a primary bone tumor or a secondary area of metastases—especially if there is cortical erosion or expansive destruction of surrounding tissues.

REFERENCES

1. Bernstein AL, Jacobs A M: Cyst and cystlike lesions of the foot. J Foot Surg 24:3–17, 1985.
2. Milgram JW: Intraosseous lipomas: Radiologic and pathologic manifestations. Radiology 167: 155–160, 1998.
3. Schatz S G, Dipaola JD, D'Agostino A, et al: Intraosseous lipoma of the calcaneus. J Foot Ankle Surg 31(4): 381–384, 1992.

PATIENT 3

A 24-year-old man with a crushed foot

A 24-year-old man relates a history of having his right foot crushed in a hydrolic jack-lift 2 days ago while at work. The patient had immediate pain and swelling and sought treatment through employee health, where x-rays revealed no fractures or dislocations of the right foot. As pain and numbness progressed, the patient sought additional medical advice.

Physical Examination: Vital signs: normal. General: mild distress. HEENT: normal. Cardiac: regular rate, no murmurs. Chest: clear breath sounds. Abdomen: soft, nontender. Extremities: nonpalpable DP pulse with a palpable posterior tibial pulse on right; 2+ nonpitting edema to the medial forefoot and arch area; ecchymosis extends from arch to hallux and first interspace. Neurological: decreased sensation (two-point discrimination, sharp and dull) dorsally, toes to ankle; all extensor tendon function intact, but increased pain with passive ROM of toe extensors.

Laboratory Findings: Radiographs of right foot: increased soft tissue density; no fractures or dislocations.

Question: What syndrome explains this patient's signs and symptoms?

5

Diagnosis: Compartment syndrome right foot

Discussion: Compartment syndromes of the upper and lower extremities are well-recognized complications of trauma. Eighty percent of compartment syndromes occur in the lower extremity. Aside from trauma, other etiologies are fracture, musculoskeletal surgery, hematoma, and infection.

Early signs and symptoms are: pain (usually out of proportion to what is expected for the clinical situation); increased pain with passive stretch of tendons in the suspected areas of disorder—the osteofascial compartments; the presence of pulses or, in severe or advanced cases, pulselessness; paresthesia, followed by hypoesthesia and anesthesia; pink (normal) capillary refill; and decreased sensation in the distribution at the posterior tibial, deep peroneal, or superficial peroneal nerves via two-point discrimination, light touch, and pin prick. Note that the most reliable indicator of the syndrome is an intracompartmental pressure > 30 mmHg as measured by a Wicks catheter.

Compartment syndrome begins with increased tissue pressure causing increased pressure on the vessel walls. This leads to increased venous pressure, a decreased arteriovenous gradient, and overall decreased local blood flow and oxygenation. After approximately 30 minutes of ischemia, paresthesia occurs. Within 2–4 hours, functional changes occur in the involved muscles, resulting in paresis. In 4–12 hours, irreversible muscle deterioration begins, and in 12+ hours, contractures form. After 24 hours marks the onset of myoglo-binuria, which, if unrecognized, can lead to acute renal failure.

Time is of the essence in diagnosing and treating compartment syndrome, as the late sequelae are permanent dysfunction and disfiguration.

Treatment consists of removing all casts and dressings and keeping the limb at heart level, as elevation creates more ischemia and interferes with venous return. Hydration is also important to help counteract the effects of myoglobinuria. In severe, progressive compartment syndrome, surgical decompression is indicated via either a single or double incision that allows adequate decompression of the medial, interosseus, central, and lateral compartments (see figure).

In the present patient, a surgical incisional release of the medial and central compartments resolved the syndrome.

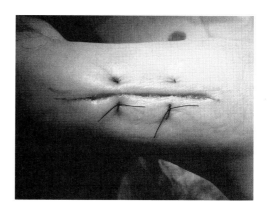

Clinical Pearls

1. Remember the 7 Ps: pain, paresthesia, paralysis, pain on passive ROM, pulses or pulselessness, and pink.
2. Compartment pressures > 30 mmHg are diagnostic of compartment syndrome.
3. Do not elevate the limb in question.
4. Hydrate the patient to prevent myoglobinuria and acute renal failure.
5. The best treatment of compartment syndrome is fasciotomy.
6. Late-stage findings are drop foot, clawing of toes, and sensory and ischemic changes.

REFERENCES

1. McGlamry E, Banks A, Downey M: Comprehensive Textbook of Foot Surgery, 2nd ed. Baltimore, MD, Williams & Wilkins, 1992.
2. Myerson M: Management of compartment syndromes of the foot. Clin Ortho v. 271, 1991.

PATIENT 4

A 56-year-old woman with shooting posterior heel pain

A 56-year-old woman presents with a 5-month history of posterior superior right heel pain. Initially, she noticed sharp, shooting pain that was remitting, but it progressed to constant tenderness approximately 3–4 weeks after the onset of initial symptoms. Irritating pain, swelling, and tenderness are present with both ambulation and nonweight-bearing, but are especially aggravated with activity. The patient denies any precipitating activity or history of trauma to the area. Conservative treatment consisted of anti-inflammatory medication, physical therapy, cam walker, and rest, with minimal relief of symptoms.

Physical Examination: Temperature 98.2° F; pulse 74; respirations 17; blood pressure 145/80. HEENT: normal. Lungs: clear. Cardiac: regular. Abdomen: nontender. Skin: normal texture/turgor/temperature. Musculoskeletal: pain on palpation of posterior superior aspect of right calcaneus and Achilles tendon at its insertion; slightly proximal, palpable osseous protuberance on superior posterior surface of right calcaneus; nontender plantar fascia or plantar medial tubercle of calcaneus; no signs of crepitus on ROM of right Achilles tendon, but positive discomfort on dorsiflexion and plantarflexion of right ankle; manual muscle testing of lower extremity—decreased plantarflexory power of the right ankle, all other muscle groups normal.

Laboratory Findings: Radiographs of right foot/ankle: mild arthritic changes in ankle with talar neck lipping, decreased calcaneal inclination angle with mild prominent posterior superior calcaneus (Haglund's deformity), prominent plantar calcaneal spur. MRI of right foot/ankle (see figure): lack of homogenicity with multiple intratendinous splits; intratendinous fluid within Achilles tendon through multiple slices on axial view of T2-weighted image; increased thickness of Achilles tendon and decreased signal intensity within the tendon approximately 2–5 cm from Achilles insertional area on T1-weighted image.

Question: What is the most likely cause of the patient's posterior superior heel pain?

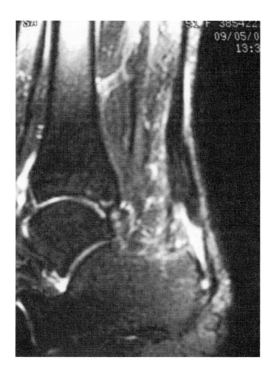

Diagnosis: Chronic Achilles tendon rupture with minor Haglund's deformity

Discussion: Posterior superior heel pain can encompass many entities. Retrocalcaneal or retro-Achilles bursitis, Haglund's deformity, Achilles tendon dysfunction or rupture, retrocalcaneal spurring or enthesopathy, and possible fracture are some of the more common entries in the differential diagnosis. A thorough history and physical, as well as plain-film radiography, bone scan, and MRI can help narrow your differential.

The diagnosis of chronic Achilles tendon tear is based on the patient's symptoms, the physical exam, and, many times, magnetic resonance imaging. There are several hypotheses regarding the cause of Achilles tendon rupture. Some of the more-recognized etiologies that have been linked to the disorder include intratendinous steroid injections, mucoid degeneration and microtears within the tendon, intensive physical training without proper warm-up, chronic tendinous inflammation or tenosynovitis, and retrocalcaneal spurring.

When the diagnosis of chronic Achilles tendon rupture is the made, the physician most then implement a treatment course. Conservative therapy is often employed first, consisting of a combination of NSAIDS, rest, physical therapy (such as phonophoresis, proprioceptive exercises, ultrasound, ice, whirlpool), accommodative padding, heel lifts, and functional orthotics. If conservative care is exhausted without any significant relief in symptoms, then surgical intervention is usually undertaken. Surgical treatment typically involves tendon repair, tenolysis, bursectomy, and excision of calcinosis and any bony prominences as deemed appropriate. Various surgical techniques and postoperative protocols that have been established and refined over the years have proven effective.

In the present patient, a repair of the Achilles was performed, along with a resection of the retrocalcaneal spur. She healed well, and the pain resolved.

Clinical Pearls

1. There are many theories regarding rupture of the Achilles tendon, but the true etiology is still unclear.

2. The Achilles tendon is different from other tendons inserting into the foot because it lacks a synovial sheath. It has a paratenon instead.

3. The Achilles tendon has an area of decreased vascularity, known as the "watershed" area. This area is approximately 2–6 cm proximal to the Achilles insertion and is particularly vulnerable to rupture.

4. MRI is very useful in determining Achilles tendon pathology, particularly in the axial and sagittal views.

5. Conservative therapy often fails to alleviate the symptoms associated with chronic Achilles tendon ruptures. Surgical intervention may be necessary.

REFERENCES

1. Clement DB, Taunton JE, Smart GW: Achilles tendonitis and peritendonitis: Etiology and treatment. Am J Sports Med 2: 179–184, 1984.
2. Maffulli N, Testa V, Capasso G: Achilles tendon rupture in athletes: Histochemistry of the triceps surae muscle. J Foot Ankle Surg 30(6): 529–533, 1991.
3. Saxena A: Surgery for chronic Achilles tendon problems. J Foot Ankle Surg 34(3): 294–300, 1995.

PATIENT 5

A 63-year-old woman with insulin-dependent diabetes and non-healing ulcers

A 63-year-old woman presents with multiple small ulcerations on the dorsum of her right foot. The bases of the ulcers are necrotic and surrounded by periwound hyperpigmented sclerotic plaque. The patient has a long history of non-healing ulcers on the dorsum of her right foot. At age 61, an erythematous papule developed in this same area. The lesion remained relatively stable for 12 months, but then began to erode and become inflamed, and she noted purulent drainage from the periphery of the lesion.

Physical Examination: Temperature 98.9° F; pulse 82; respirations 18; blood pressure 188/89. Skin: otherwise normal. HEENT: normal. Lungs: clear. Cardiac: normal. Abdomen: nontender. Lower extremity: nonpalpable dorsalis pedis pulse on the right foot, all other pulses weakly palpable; diffuse tenderness noted over entire dorsal aspect of right foot; necrotic base of ulcers, fibrinous wound edges, periwound hyperpigmented sclerotic plaques surrounded by erythema (see figure).

Laboratory Findings: WBC 11,000/μl, hemoglobin 10 g/dl, Hct 26.9%, platelets 300,000/μl. Urinalysis normal.

Question: What is the etiology of the patient's ulcers?

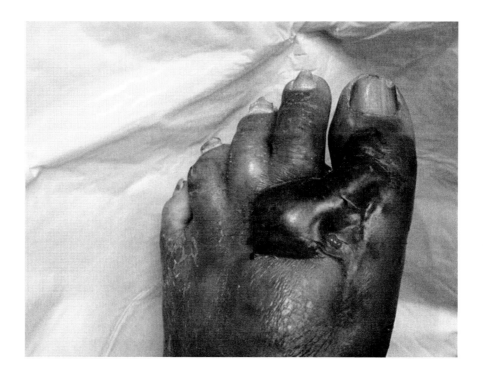

Diagnosis: Necrobiosis lipoidica diabeticorum

Discussion: Necrobiosis lipoidica, according to Muller and Winkelmann, is a degenerative disease of dermal connective tissue characterized clinically by an inflammatory, pretibial, sclerodermatous plaque that is often associated with diabetes mellitus. Necrobiosis lipoidica is not directly related to hyperglycemia, but rather is a result of deposits of immunoglobulins and complement in the vessel walls. Ullman and Dahl suggest that the pathogenesis of necrobiosis is an immune complex vasculitis. This is supported by Handelsman, who believes that a glycoprotein is deposited in the blood vessel walls and between the collagen bundles, and that trauma often determines the site of necrobiosis.

Pathological findings of necrobiosis include ill-defined areas of fibrosis associated with granulomatous infiltrate with lymphocytes and plasma cells. Histologically there is palisading of histiocytes about the necrobiotic areas, especially in diabetic patients, who are more likely to have intimal thickening and perivascular fibrosis of the middle and lower dermal vessels close to the necrobiotic areas. Deposition of fat is also seen in the necrobiotic areas.

Necrobiosis lipoidica usually begins as an erythematous papule or nodule. The lesion becomes a shiny, waxy, or yellowish-red sclerotic plaque. The central portion of the lesion becomes slightly scaly, atrophic, and depressed, and ulceration may develop. The most common location for necrobiotic lesions is the pretibial region. They may also be manifested on the thighs, popliteal areas, and dorsum of feet and arms. The lesions tend to be multiple, bilateral, and symmetrical. Misdiagnosis can occur because of variation in size, shape, location, or inflammatory degenerative changes.

The differential diagnosis of necrobiosis lipoidica should include sarcoid, granuloma annulare, stasis dermatitis, posttraumatic fibrosis with hemosiderosis, rheumatoid nodules, erythema induratum, ecthyma, nodular panniculitis, and xanthoma.

Treatment of the lesion is quite controversial. However, most agree that although this lesion is commonly seen in diabetic patients, complete control of the diabetes does not affect the course of the lesion.

The present patient had necrobiosis lipoidica diabeticorum that was secondarily infected by methycillian-resistant *Staphylococcus aureus.* The patient underwent a popliteal-dorsalis pedis bypass to increase blood flow to the involved area. The wounds were debrided intraoperatively, and a full course of vancomycin was completed. The patient went on to heal uneventfully.

Clinical Pearls

1. Necrobiosis lipoidica occurs in both diabetic and nondiabetic patients.
2. Development is not directly related to hyperglycemia.
3. Spontaneous resolution of lesions can occur after years of persistance.
4. Necrobiosis is most commonly found in the pretibial region; however, it can occur on the thigh, popliteal fossa, dorsum of foot or forearm, and other areas.

REFERENCE

Campbell DR: Diabetic vascular disease. In Frykberg R: The High-Risk Foot in Diabetes Mellitus. New York, Churchill Livingstone, 1991, pp 33–38.

PATIENT 6

A 46-year-old man with a cyanotic hallux and fifth toe

A 46-year-old man presents with a 3-day history of increased cyanosis of the hallux and the fifth toe plantarly, increased swelling, and eruptions of multiple bullae. The patient has a long history of drug and alcohol abuse and was recently living in an unheated, abandoned house. He was brought to the hospital by his mother for exacerbation of herpes zoster with secondary bacterial infection on his buttocks and bilateral thighs. The patient had lost his third and fourth toes to frostbite 3 years earlier.

Physical Examination: Temperature 100.6° F; pulse 65; respirations 15; blood pressure 100/68. Skin: large eruptions of herpes zoster effecting multiple dermatomes on the back, buttocks, and posterior thighs. HEENT: normal. Lungs: clear. Cardiac: normal. Abdomen: non-tender. Lower extremity: pulses palpable in dorsalis pedis and posterior tibial arteries; hallux and lateral digits cold, with cyanosis; increased pedal edema; multiple bullae with clear fluid plantarly under digits (see figure); decreased epicritic, sharp-dull, and protective sensation bilaterally.

Laboratory Findings: WBC 9000/μl, hemoglobin 11 g/dl, Hct 29.9%, platelets 300,000/μl. Urinalysis: normal.

Question: What is the etiology of the patient's pedal presentation?

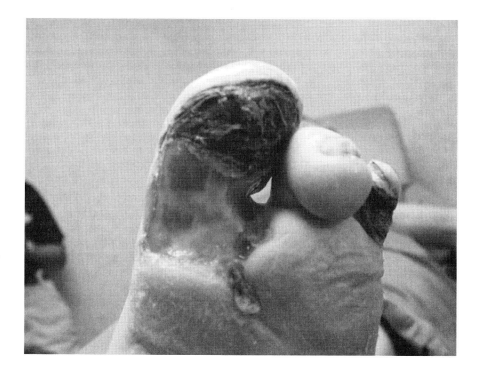

Diagnosis: Frostbite

Discussion: Frostbite is an injury that results from exposing the body to temperatures of 0 degrees or colder; peripheral tissue freeze at the cellular level. Hayes et al suggest that this leads to inflammation, free radical–induced tissue damage, vascular deficiencies, platelet function abnormalities, and ischemic-reperfusion injury.

The pathophysiology of frostbite has been attributed to two distinct mechanisms according to Weatherly-White et al: (1) cellular death that occurs at the time of exposure, and (2) deterioration and necrosis attributable to progressive dermal ischemia.

Clinical manifestations of frostbite have been categorized according to Murphy et al into four degrees. **First-degree** frostbite presents with a centralized white plaque that is numb and surrounded by erythema. **Second-degree** injury has blister with a clear or milky fluid and is surrounded by erythema and edema. **Third-degree** injury is characterized by hemorrhagic blisters that result in hard, black eschars 2 weeks later. **Fourth-degree** injury produces complete necrosis and tissue loss. However, this staging does not help in predicting the extent of tissue loss.

Radiographic imaging can aid the physician in predicting the level of demarcation or tissue loss. Plain radiographs can demonstrate soft tissue swelling in early stages, and osteoporosis and periostitis in later stages. Gralino suggests that arteriography can demonstrate the slowing of flow and occlusions that occur, but does not adequately clarify the level of injury. Bone scan, according to Ikawa, has now become the standard imaging study in the first few days of injury and can be used to guide a surgeon and allow earlier debridement of damaged areas. However, it does not show "clear-cut" level of demarcation. MR angiography has been suggested to aid in the accuracy of determining the level of demarcation; however, no studies have yet been published.

According to Murphy et al, there are **three phases of treatment** for frostbite. First, in the prethaw phase, it is imperative to protect the area involved from mechanical trauma or from slowed rewarming. In the second phase, rewarming, it is important to rapidly rewarm the involved areas. Placing the involved extremities in a 40- to 42-degree waterbath with hexachlorophene or betadine for 15 to 30 minutes is the best way to accomplish this task. Active motion of the involved part is also recommended.

McCauley et al have recommended a protocol for the final, postthaw phase. Paramount are suppression of local and systemic thromboxane, adequate analgesia, and prevention of infection. Ibuprofen (a systemic inhibitor of thromboxane) and aloe vera (a topical antithromboxane), combined with penicillin and a vasodilator such as oxpentifylline, can improve tissue survival. Debridement of clear blisters, which represent superficial injury, can reduce further contact with the high levels of prostaglandin F2 and thromboxane A2 in the exudate. Hemorrhagic blisters that represent damage to the dermal plexus may benefit from aspiration; however, many believe they should be left intact.

The current patient presented several days after injury; thus the prethaw and rapid rewarming phases could not be initiated. His clear blisters were debrided, and since prevention of infection was a priority, he was placed on cefazolin. The patient is scheduled for continued follow-up appointments to watch for level of demarcation.

Clinical Pearls

1. Management of injury should include:
   - Protection of the involved area prior to rewarming
   - Rapid rewarming in 40- to 42-degree Celsius waterbath with hexachlorophene or betadine for 15 to 30 minutes
   - Triple therapy with ibuprofen, aloe vera, and penicillin.
2. Bone scan can aid in early determination of the level of demarcation.
3. Complete demarcation of the involved extremity should be acquired before surgical debridement is attempted—barring signs of infection.

REFERENCE
Washburn B: Frostbite: What is it, how to prevent it, emergency treatment. New Eng J Med 266:974, 1962.

PATIENT 7

A 46-year-old woman with a hot and swollen foot

A 46-year-old woman presents to the emergency department with a red, hot, and swollen foot that is causing her pain. She states that over the course of 7 days the foot became massively edematous, red, and very warm. She denies any history of trauma. The patient has a past medical history significant for insulin-dependent diabetes mellitus and hypertension.

Physical Examination: Temperature 97.9° F; pulse 63; respirations 16; blood pressure 100/56. Skin: normal. HEENT: normal. Chest: clear. Cardiac: normal. Abdomen: nontender. Lower extremity: nonpalpable dorsalis pedis and posterior tibial pulses on left foot secondary to massive edema, audible with Doppler; left foot warm in comparison with contralateral side; grade 2 pitting edema from distal left foot to middle third of left leg. Skin: large bullae on plantar distal left foot from submetatarsals 3 to 5; small hyperkeratotic lesion with hemorrhagic central area at submetatarsal 2.

Laboratory Findings: WBC 13,000/μl, Hg 12.1, Hct 29.3, platelet 200,000/μl. Urinalysis: normal.

Question: What is the etiology of this foot disorder?

Diagnosis: Puncture wound with foreign body

Discussion: A variety of foreign bodies are common following a puncture wound. Serious complications can develop if proper diagnosis and treatment are not established. Complications may include osteomyelitis, abscess, epidermoid inclusion cysts, septic arthritis, gas gangrene, sepsis, and possibly loss of limb or life.

Diagnosis of foreign body can be made with careful history and physical examination. Radiographic evaluation can reveal all metal fragments and most glass regardless of lead content. Tandberg confirmed that all glass is visible radiographically because the density of the glass is greater than that of the surrounding tissue. He studied 66 types of glass and concluded that heavy metals or pigments are not required for radioopacity. Xeroradiography, ultrasonography, CT, and MR imaging can be helpful in defining small pieces of glass.

Detection of wood with standard radiographs is difficult. Studies by Charney and Woesner compared the use of standard radiography and xeroradiography. The results of Charney's work contradicted that of Woesner. Position of the fragment was determined to be the most important factor for visualization. Wood is best seen with MRI. The inflammatory capsule produced by the body in response to the foreign wood fragment is seen easily on T2-weighted images.

The first step in management of foreign bodies is removal of the offensive agent. This can be accomplished at beside if the wound is superficial, or in the operating room if necessary. The puncture tract should be reopened and explored. All devitalized tissue and foreign bodies should be removed. If an abscess is present, surgical incision and drainage are required. The area should then be x-rayed again to assure that all foreign substances were removed. Pack the wound to allow drainage and prevent premature closure. Cultures should be taken at the time of surgical debridement to identify the causative agent and allow for proper selection of antibiotic therapy.

The second step is selecting the appropriate antibiotics until final culture results can be obtained. The most common infective agents in a puncture wound with cellulitis are *Staphylococcus aureus,* alpha-hemolytic streptococci, *Staphylococcus epidermidis, Escherichia coli,* and Proteus. The most common organism found in puncture wounds with osteomyelitis is *Pseudomonas aeruginosa.* Cefazolin, ampicillin/sulbactam, ticarcillin/clavulanic acid, or clindamycin for puncture wounds associated with cellulitis are recommended. If osteomyelitis is suspected, ceftazidime or ciprofloxacin are excellent choices.

In the present patient, glass embedded in the base of the wound probed deeply to the dorsal surface of the foot. An abscess was located plantarly from the second metatarsal to the fifth. The patient was started on empiric antibiotics (injected cefazolin and metronidazole) and taken to the operating room for immediate incision and drainage. At the time of surgery, a small piece of glass was removed from the wound. The area was packed open, and the patient received dressing changes twice a day. Her culture results came back positive for coagulase-negative staphylococci (multi-drug resistant) and enterococci. The patient's antibiotics were changed to vancomycin for a 2-week course. She went on to heal uneventfully.

Clinical Pearls

1. Once the diagnosis of osteomyelitis with puncture wound is made, the treatment must be swift.

2. Superficial wounds can be treated with local wound care. Deep wounds should be completed explored and debrided. When in doubt, open it up.

3. Convert the contaminated wound to a clean wound.

4. Prevent tetanus; consider one dose of tetanus immune globulin for all wounds that are suspicious and not clean.

REFERENCES

1. Charney DB, Manzi JA, et al: Nonmetallic foreign bodies in the foot: Radiography versus xeroradiography. J Foot Surg 25:44–49, 1986.
2. Fitzgerald R, Cowan J: Puncture wounds of the foot. Orthop Clin North Am 6:965–972, 1975.
3. Johanson P: Pseudomonas infections of the foot following puncture wounds. JAMA 204:170–172, 1968.
4. Joseph WS: Handbook of Lower Extremity Infections. New York, Churchill Livingstone, 1990.

PATIENT 8

A 22-year-old man with pain in his third toe

A 22-year-old man presents with pain in his left third digit. He was jumping off a diving board when he felt a "snap" in this toe. He had pain immediately following this sensation and had difficulty moving the toe. The patient is healthy, with no past medical history.

Physical Examination: Temperature 98.6° F, pulse 65, respirations 15, blood pressure 100/68. Lower extremity: pulses palpable bilaterally, left third digit slightly edematous and erythematous; pain on palpation of distal aspect of third proximal phalanx; pain with range of motion of proximal interphalangeal joint.

Laboratory Findings: WBC 5000/μl, Hg 16, Hct 36.9, platelets 300,000/μl. Urinalysis: normal.

Question: What is the etiology of the patient's pain?

Diagnosis: Enchondroma with pathologic fracture

Discussion: An <u>enchondroma</u> is a tumor that develops in the medullary cavity and is composed of lobules of hyaline cartilage. The neoplasm is usually discovered in the third to fourth decade of life. It is seen equally in men and women. Solitary enchondromas are usually asymptomatic and are therefore diagnosed as an incidental finding on radiograph or bone scan. Resnick suggests that pain associated with a lesion can be suggestive of malignant transformation—a complication that is more commonly noted in the long tubular bones.

According to a study by Arata et al., enchondromas represent about 3% percent of biopsy-analyzed primary bone tumors. Resnick and Marco et al state that approximately 40–65% of solitary enchondromas occur in the hands or the feet. It is one of the most common tumors found in the foot. Arata et al. suggest, however, that the most common sites of involvement in order of decreasing frequency are diaphysis, metadiaphysis of the femur (40%), humurus, tibia, and short tubular bones of the hands and feet. Less common sites include the ribs, radius, fibula, ulna, and pelvis. Some enchondromas lead to osseous expansion (enchondroma protuberans) that simulates the appearance of an osteochondroma.

Radiographic examination, as described by Marco et al, reveals a well-defined, medullary lesion with stippled calcification, a lobulated contour, and endosteal scalloping. Lesions may demonstrate cortical expansion and pathologic fracture. MRI reveals a well-circumscribed lesion of low signal intensity in T1-weighted images and of high signal intensity in T2-weighted images. Calcifications may appear as regions of low signal intensity.

Most enchondromas consist microscopically of lobules of hyaline-type cartilage. They also contain calcified regions in which the cells may appear degenerative or necrotic.

Marco et al state that enchondromas in the small tubular bones of the hands and feet rarely transform into chondrosarcomas, which are the usual result of malignancy. Malignant transformation is more likely in enchondromas in the long tubular or flat bones. Indications of malignant transformation include an enlarging radiolucent area, cortical expansion, pathologic fracture, soft tissue mass, and disappearance of pre-existing calcification.

The present patient sustained a pathologic fracture of a previously undiagnosed enchondroma. He was taken to the operating room where the dorsal cortex of the third proximal phalanx was penetrated by a curette. The enchondroma was evacuated and sent for frozen section, which demonstrated a benign cartilaginous tumor. A burr was used to remove any remaining aspects of the cartilaginous tumor form the inner lining. The bone was flushed and packed with corticocancellous bone chips. The patient went on to heal uneventfully.

Clinical Pearls

1. Enchondromas are found equally in men and women, generally in the third and fourth decades of life.

2. Enchondromas are most often asymptomatic.

3. These tumors are most commonly found in the hands and feet, but are also seen in the femur, tibia, and humerus.

4. Enchondromas that are painful or sustain a fracture should be biopsied to rule out malignant transformation.

REFERENCES

1. Arata MA, Peterson JA, Dahlin DC: Pathologic fracture through non-ossifying fibromas. J Bone Joint Surg 63A:980–988, 1981.
2. Marco RA, Gitelis S, et al: Cartilage tumors: Evaluation and treatment. J Am Acad Ortho Surg 8(5):292–304, 2000.
3. Resnick CS, Levine AM, et al: Case Report 522: Concurrent adjacent osteochondroma and enchondroma. Skel Radiol 18(1):66–69, 1989.

PATIENT 9

A 33-year-old woman with a painful right ankle

A 33-year-old woman presents with a chief complaint of pain on the lateral aspect of her right ankle. The pain has been present for about 2 weeks and had a relatively acute onset. The patient, who is an avid runner, stated that she was in the middle of a 10-mile run when she began to experience "significant pain" in her outer ankle, which prevented her from finishing the run. Currently, she is unable to run because the pain is too intense during exercise. The patient's past medical history is unremarkable, and her only medication is oral contraceptives.

Physical Examination: Vital signs: normal. Skin: mild localized edema at lateral right ankle; no ecchymosis or open lesions present. Musculoskeletal: tenderness on palpation of right lateral malleolus and right distal fibula; tenderness on palpation of peroneal tendons, posterior to right lateral malleolus. ROM: normal right ankle, subtalar, and midtarsal joints; tenderness on resistance against eversion of subtalar joint. No gross orthopedic malalignment noted.

Laboratory Findings: Radiographs: no occult fractures or other osseous lesions of distal right fibula. MRI: distal third of right fibula included both a linear decreased intensity on T1-weighted image and a localized increased intensity on T2 in same area.

Question: What is the likely cause of the patient's right ankle pain?

Diagnosis: Stress fracture of right fibula

Discussion: Stress fractures are fairly common clinical entities encountered in podiatric medical practice. They are generally the result of a repetitive, sub-threshold amount of load on a bone. The load, which represents abnormal stress on an otherwise normal bone, can be a result of ground reactive forces or cyclic tension from tendinous and ligamentous attachments. Similar in outcome but different in cause are insufficiency fractures, which relate to normal stresses placed upon an abnormal bone. Insufficiency fractures are seen in patients with osteoporosis, osteomalacia, Paget's disease, and other metabolic bone disorders.

Stress fractures can be seen in the metatarsals, calcaneus, fibula, tibia, femur, navicular, sesamoid, and other bones of the lower extremity and, less frequently, in some bones of the upper extremity. They generally occur in the physically active, especially in runners. Several factors contribute to the development of stress fractures. The most common factor is training error; for example, a significant increase in training distances or a decrease in intervals between long runs. More intense training allows little time for the affected bone to adapt physiologically to the increased stresses placed upon it. Other factors are rigid running surfaces, poor shoe gear, and poor physical fitness. Anatomic malalignments such as limb length discrepancies, hyperpronation, and rigid cavus feet also may lead to stress fractures.

Diagnosis can at times be a difficult problem, but several signs and symptoms are helpful. The patient's history usually includes an insidious onset of symptoms while training. The pain is usually relieved with cessation of activity. Further questioning of the patient may uncover recent changes in training habits, such as higher mileage, different running surfaces, or new sneakers. Physical exam may reveal an abnormal gait, pain on palpation over the affected area, and localized warmth.

Confirmation of stress fracture generally requires a radiograph, bone scan, or MRI. Recent stress fractures may not appear on x-ray, as osseous changes require 2–3 weeks to register on film. Some radiographic signs include periosteal reaction, a small break in the bone cortex, and/or a focal area of sclerosis. Stress fractures within the cortical portion of long bone usually show a periosteal reaction; in the metaphyseal portion, which is made of cancellous bone, they show a sclerotic line.

Patients with a suspicious clinical presentation but no evidence of stress fracture on conventional x-ray require more sensitive and specific testing. Bone scans remain a good option for diagnosing a stress fracture. They are highly sensitive for bone turnover and are positive long before an x-ray. They will show an increased area of uptake in the area of the fracture. Bone scans are sensitive but not specific for fracture, and positive results could be due to malignancy and bone infection.

MRI has become a more popular modality for diagnosing stress fracture. In the present patient, MRI was chosen because of her soft tissue symptoms, including peroneal tendonitis, which can be ruled out using this modality. In this case, the T2-weighted image showed increased intensity within the medullary canal of the fibula, and the T1 image showed a transverse line of hypointensity with a cortical break in the same area.

Treatment of stress fractures is much easier when an early diagnosis is made. Early on, simple rest may go a long way toward relieving the symptoms. This, along with ice and NSAIDs, can be sufficient to allow the bone to heal. If a later diagnosis is made, immobilization of the affected area may be required. Some bones affected by a stress fracture may require more aggressive therapy, such as surgical fixation, because of their poor healing ability; these include the base of the fifth metatarsal, the navicular, and the scaphoid in the hand. Once the stress fracture is healed, it is imperative for the athlete to change the training habits that led to the fracture.

Clinical Pearls

1. Radiographs may be negative immediately following the injury. Two to three weeks later, a periosteal reaction may be visualized.

2. Bone scan is sensitive, but not specific.

3. MRI shows a linear decrease in intensity on T1 and increased intensity on T2-weighted images.

REFERENCES

1. McBryde AM: Stress fractures in athletes. J Sports Med 3:212–17, 1975.
2. Santi M, Sartoris DJ, Resnick D: Magnetic resonance imaging in the diagnosis of metatarsal stress fractures. J Foot Surg 27: 172–77, 1988.
3. Taunton JE, et.al: Lower extremity stress fracture in athletes. Phys Sports Med 9: 77–83, 1981.
4. Wilson E, Katz F: Stress fractures: An analysis of 250 consecutive cases. Radiology 92: 481–86, 1969.

PATIENT 10

A 56-year-old man with a traumatic injury to his ankle

A 56-year-old man presents to the emergency department (ED) immediately following a traumatic incident to his right ankle. The patient was walking on the sidewalk when his right foot hit a steel elevation in the sidewalk. His was body propelled forward while his foot remained planted. He is currently unable to bear weight on that foot. The patient's medical history is noncontributory, but he does mention a right ankle sprain 40 years earlier.

Physical Examination: Skin: moderate swelling; no ecchymosis. Musculoskeletal: pain on palpation to anterior aspect of ankle joint, which extended to both malleoli; pain on attempted range of motion (ROM). Due to severity of pain, talar tilt and anterior drawer tests not performed.

Laboratory Findings: Radiographs: increased soft tissue density at anterior aspect of ankle joint; avulsion flecks off of lateral malleolus; incidental anterior ankle joint arthritis with spur formation. No overt fractures to ankle, no osteochondral lesions noticed, and no dislocations. Ankle joint in good alignment, and medial clear space normal.

Course: The patient was placed in a Jones' compression cast and told to take ibuprofen for the pain and inflammation. He was also informed about the principles of rest, ice, compression, and elevation. Finally, he was given crutches, with the direction to be nonweight-bearing until his follow-up appointment with his podiatrist. The patient returned 1.5 weeks later using crutch assistance. He admitted to removing the compression cast 2 days after its application due to discomfort. At that time, he had swelling and ecchymosis about the ankle joint, mostly lateral. There was continuation of pain on ROM of the ankle joint and with supination of the subtalar joint. An MRI was ordered.

MRI Findings: Partial tears of anterior and posterior talofibular ligaments, with joint effusion through these defects. Calcaneal fibular ligament could not be visualized on any of MRI cuts, and extent of pathology could not be appreciated. Deltoid ligaments intact; no abnormalities of tibiotalar and subtalar joints.

Question: What is the best treatment option for this injury?

Answer: Removal of bone flecks and reattachment of ligaments

Discussion: Ankle trauma, which displays as ankle pain, edema, and ecchymosis, is very common. Studies have shown that up to 32% of patients with lateral ankle trauma have recurrences; thus, there is a need for lateral ankle stabilization and fixation. Awareness of the angles formed by the orientation of the ligaments and their relation to the ankle and subtalar joint axes is crucial for understanding the mechanics of ankle sprains.

As the foot moves through its range of motion during gait, the anterior talofibular ligament is mostly used to resist inversion when the ankle is plantarflexed and the ligament is parallel to the fibula. The calcaneofibular ligament, being the only lateral collateral ligament to pass the ankle joint and subtalar joint, lies nearly parallel to the subtalar joint axis and allows unrestricted motion in the subtalar

joint. The more these ligaments are sprained, the weaker they become, and they will not be able to resist the forces coming across the ankle and subtalar joints. Intraoperative repair is required for both recurrence of ankle sprains and a single traumatic event obliterating the ankle joint ligaments.

In the present patient, arthroscopy showed acute synovitis between the inferior tibial surface and the lateral malleolus and cartilage damage within the right ankle joint. The anterior talofibular ligament of the lateral ankle joint was partially torn, and the calcaneal fibular and posterior fibular ligaments could not be visualized. There were avulsion fractures off of both the anterior talofibular and calcaneal fibular ligaments. The avulsed pieces of bone were removed, and the ligaments were reattached using PEBA anchors.

Clinical Pearls

1. When examining patients with ankle injuries, take extra time to carefully scrutinize the ankle joint for ligament tears and fractures. Also perform a complete examination to rule out any fractures or dislocations.

2. Radiographic evidence of bone flecks inferior to the lateral malleolus is highly suggestive of avulsion fractures in the ligaments about the ankle joint.

3. MRI studies are not always completely accurate and should not be the only modality used for diagnosis. Take into account the mechanism of injury, the clinical findings, and the radiographic studies to help corroborate your findings.

4. If surgery is needed, intraoperative visualization of the injury is the best way to make your final diagnosis.

REFERENCES

1. Hamilton W: The modified Bronstrom procedure for lateral ankle instability. Foot Ankle 14(1): 1–7, 1993.
2. Perlman M: Inversion lateral ankle trauma: Differential diagnosis, review of the literature, and prospective study. J Foot Surg 26(2): 95–129, 1987.

PATIENT 11

A 44-year-old woman with right foot pain of insidious onset

A 44-year-old woman presents to the office with a complaint of pain in the dorsal aspect of her right foot for a period of 2 months. She relates a somewhat insidious onset, as well as radiation of pain and some occasional tingling into her third and fourth toes. The pain is generally present while the patient is ambulating, and it feels better when she rests. She was seen at an emergency department approximately 2 weeks prior, with severe pain in the same foot. Radiographs taken at that time revealed no osseous deformity. Past medical history is significant for depression. Her only medication is Prozac. The patient is allergic to codeine, penicillin, and sulfa drugs. She denies tobacco and alcohol use.

Physical Examination: General: no apparent distress. Lower extremities: bilateral palpable pedal pulses; normal capillary refill time; no edema of the right foot. Skin: no open lesions; normal color/turgor/texture; no erythema. Musculoskeletal: palpation of right foot caused pain between 2nd and 3rd metatarsals just proximal to metatarsal heads, radiating into 2nd and 3rd toes; lateral compression of medial and lateral foot caused pain in second interspace; palpation at base of 2nd metatarsal and plantarflexion of Lisfranc's joint also caused pain. Neurologic: decreased sensation to light touch and pain along lateral aspect of 2nd digit and medial aspect of 3rd digit.

Laboratory Findings: Radiograph (see figure) and MRI of right foot: bone defect at base of second metatarsal; false motion when put through ROM under fluoroscopy; sclerosed bone ends developing at base of second metatarsal.

Question: What is the cause or causes of the patient's pain?

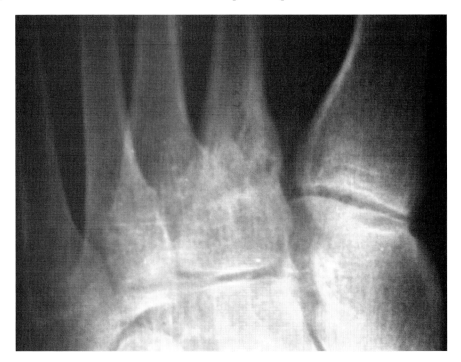

Diagnosis: Neuroma and fracture nonunion of 2nd metatarsal

Discussion: The initial impression on first examining this patient led the physician to lean toward a diagnosis of neuroma of the 2nd interspace. However, palpation of the 2nd metatarsal directly revealed pain that was more consistent with a stress or occult fracture of the 2nd metatarsal. The x-ray of the foot demonstrated a sclerotic area and a periosteal reaction at the base of the 2nd metatarsal. Because of the possibility of a concomitant neuroma, it was decided that MRI would be the best choice to visualize both the neuroma and the metatarsal fracture. The MRI showed increased signal intensity within the marrow of the 2nd metatarsal base on the T2-weighted image and an enlarged interdigital nerve in the 2nd interspace.

With over 2 million bone fractures in the U.S. each year, there is about 5% incidence of nonunions and even more delayed unions. There is not a distinct line clinically and radiographically that delineates a nonunion from a delayed union. Generally, the diagnosis of a **delayed union** is made when a fracture has not advanced at an average rate of healing for a particular type and location of fracture. This time frame is usually 3–6 months, but is variable depending on the bone and type of fracture. A **nonunion** diagnosis requires evidence either clinically or on x-ray that healing has ceased and union across the fracture site is highly unlikely. The FDA has further classified a nonunion as a fracture that has failed to completely heal after a minimum of 9 months, and healing has not progressed radiographically for a period of 3 months.

Delayed union and nonunion can be due to both local and systemic factors. Systemic factors include the patient's nutritional status, activity level, and even tobacco use, which has been shown to have a very detrimental effect on bone healing. Local factors include motion at the fracture site, inadequate fixation, open fractures, comminuted fractures, and impaired blood supply.

Nonunions have been divided into two types based on the viability of the fracture ends. First is the *hypervascular* (or hypertrophic) type, in which the bone end is viable and capable of healing. This is different from the *avascular* (or atrophic) type, which has a nonviable bone end and no chance of biologic reaction. Hypertrophic nonunions can be further divided into the elephant foot, horsehoof, and oligotrophic types, and avascular nonunions are separated into the comminuted, torsion-wedge, defect, and atrophic types. These subdivisions are based on the blood supply—or lack thereof—supplying the bone ends.

Treatment of delayed unions in most cases can be as simple as immobilization of the fracture fragments. Electrical stimulation to accelerate the union has become popular when immobilization is insufficient to complete the consolidation. The placement of a bone stimulator causes a steady-state potential around the bone fragments, with the electronegative side stimulating osteogenesis.

Nonunions require a more aggressive treatment protocol because they have little or no chance of healing due to a dysvascular state. Such treatment is generally surgical in nature. Because the bone ends are dysvascular, they must be resected and then rigidly fixated to have any chance of healing. The repair generally requires some type of bone grafting to maintain the length of the repaired bone. Bone grafting techniques vary greatly (e.g., inlay bone grafts, onlay bone grafts). Once the procedure is completed, the repaired bone must be completely immobilized, and a bone stimulator is used to hasten consolidation. This procedure can take up to 4–6 months for complete healing.

The present patient underwent surgical resection of the dysvascular bone ends; a bone graft was placed between the two ends; and the area was immobilized with internal fixation. She was placed in a below-knee cast and was instructed to remain non-weight bearing for a total of 6 weeks. The patient went on to heal uneventfully.

Clinical Pearls

1. A nonunion is characterized by:
   A bone defect
   False motion
   Sclerosis of bone ends
   Rounding and mushrooming of bone ends
   Sealing of bone ends with compact bone.
2. Contraindications to the use of electrostimulation in the treatment of nonunions are:
   Synovial pseudoarthrosis
   Bone gap greater than half the diameter of the bone
   Bone gap greater than 1 cm
   Uncontrollable motion

REFERENCE
Brighton CT: Principle of fracture healing. Instr Course Lect 33:60, 1984.

PATIENT 12

A 60-year-old woman with a continually aching arch

A 60-year-old woman presents with a complaint of increasing tenderness in the medial aspect of her right ankle for a period of 3 months. The pain occasionally radiates distally into her foot, and generally increases while ambulating and during prolonged periods of activity. She relates no antecedent trauma that led to the onset of the pain. Further questioning reveals that she noticed a progressive flattening of the arch over the past several months. There has been no treatment to date, except for acetaminophen for the pain, which provided little relief. Past medical history includes hypertension and acid reflux; medications included metoprolol and omeprazole. She has no known drug allergies, and her only previous surgery was right foot bunionectomy without complication.

Physical Examination: General: no apparent distress. Lower Extremities: palpable pedal pulses bilaterally; normal capillary fill time, with some mild edema along medial aspect of right ankle. Skin: no ecchymosis; no open lesions; color, turgor, and texture normal. Musculoskeletal: considerable tenderness along course of posterior from just behind medial malleolous to its insertion at navicular; normal ROM at ankle joint and subtalar and midtarsal joints; manual muscle testing revealed all groups full strength, except some weakness of foot and pain on resistance against inversion; abducted forefoot on rearfoot, especially on right foot; positive heel rise test with obvious inability to rise up on toes. Neurologic: all sensation grossly intact; negative Tinel's sign in tarsal tunnel.

Laboratory Findings: MRI: thickening of tibialis posterior tendon; increased signal circumferentially, with tendon sheath effusion; increased intratendinous signal. Radiographs (lateral view, see figure): loss in longitudinal arch, with first ray elevatus and break in cyma line; on plantarflexion of talus, calcaneal inclination approached parallel weight-bearing surface; no osteoarthritic findings.

Question: What is causing the medial ankle pain?

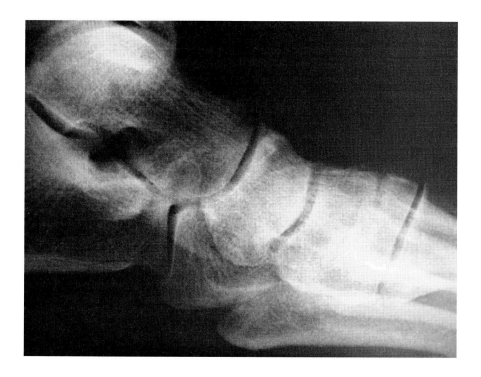

Diagnosis: Posterior tibial tendon dysfunction

Discussion: Posterior tibial (PT) tendon dysfunction has been diagnosed more frequently over the past several years. Previously, it was commonly misdiagnosed or at least under-diagnosed. A recent surge in published articles about this disorder has led to more ready recognition of its signs and symptoms.

The tendon's main function is help resist and slow rearfoot eversion upon heel strike during the stance phase of gait. As the foot progresses into mid-stance, the tendon helps lock the midtarsal joint and begins contracting to cause subtalar joint inversion. Finally, in the propulsive phase of gait the tendon accelerates subtalar joint inversion ends in heel lift. So, simply put, the posterior tibial tendon is the main inverter of the foot and is largely responsible for maintaining arch height.

There has been some controversy as to the cause of PT tendon dysfunction. It generally involves a degeneration of the tendon from a multitude of causes, each of which is usually multifactorial in nature. Some structural abnormalities, alone or in combination, which may lead to PT tendon dysfunction include an accessory navicular, rigid or flexible flatfoot, and equinus. These disorders, along with a possible zone of relative dysvascularity within the tendon between the medial malleolus and the tendon insertion, lead to degeneration within the tendon. As the tendon degenerates it begins to slowly elongate and eventually loses mechanical advantage. This loss of mechanical advantage allows the peroneus brevis to gain advantage and causes loss of arch height and midtarsal joint break.

Various classifications and staging systems have been proposed for the progression of the deformity. **Stage 1** is considered an asymptomatic period, during which the patient has nothing more than an underlying structural or anatomic abnormality that predisposes him or her to the development of PT tendon dysfunction. As the patient progresses into **stage 2,** symptoms develop that bring them to your office. Symptoms include tendinitis, some effusion behind the medial malleolus, and progression of a flat foot deformity. The patient will have tenderness along the course of the tendon, abduction of the forefoot, and failure to successfully rise up on the toes on one side. **Stage 3** is similar to stage 2, but with more disabling symptoms and greater degeneration within the tendon (e.g., longitudinal tears or partial ruptures). Finally, in **stage 4,** the patient begins to experience joint adaptation and functional disability.

Diagnosis can generally be made from the patient's history and a good clinical exam. Radiographs can be useful to assess joint adaptations in later stages of dysfunction and are useful in surgical planning. The MRI has become a useful tool to assess the pathology within the tendon, determining whether a simple tenosynovitis exists or whether the dysfunction has progressed to midsubstance tears and partial ruptures. MRI also may aid in surgical planning.

Treatment is generally based on the stage of dysfunction. Mild stage 1 dysfunction in some patients can be treated conservatively. The underlying biomechanical abnormality must be controlled to prevent further progression of the deformity. This is generally accomplished with some type of orthotic device with a high degree of varus posting. NSAIDs and physical therapy may have some benefit as well. Once the dysfunction progresses into the later stages, surgery becomes the only viable option. Surgical intervention (see figure) starts with direct tendon repair and progresses to tendon transfers and finally to bony reconstruction, including calcaneal osteotomies and subtalar arthroereisis procedures, with the last step being a triple arthrodesis.

Early and accurate diagnosis is paramount to prevent progression of deformity into the later stages of posterior tibial tendon dysfunction. The present patient had direct surgical repair of the tendon. A synovectomy was performed along with repair of the longitudinal tears that were found intraoperatively. The patient was immobilized in a short leg cast for a period of 4 weeks. Upon removal of the cast, she was provided custom-molded orthoses, and healed uneventfully.

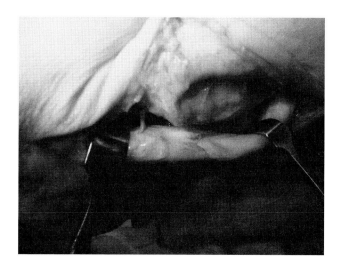

Clinical Pearls

1. In the early stages of posterior tibial tendon dysfunction, patients describe an ache along the inner side of the foot, with a moderate amount of warmth between the malleolus and the navicular.

2. When looking directly at the foot from behind, you will note the too-many-toes sign—the foot is abducted, and the toes are seen laterally.

3. The patient has difficulty standing on the toes and usually is surprised not to have noticed it earlier.

4. Simply resisting active inversion in the nonweight-bearing position usually elicits pain along the PT tendon.

5. MRI can show intrasubstance tears even in the early stages.

REFERENCES

1. Rosenberg ZS, Cheung Y: Rupture of the posterior tibial tendon: CT and MRI with surgical correlation. Radiology 169:229–235, 1988.
2. Sartoris DJ, Resnick D: Magnetic resonance imaging of tendons in the foot and ankle. J Foot Surg 28:370–377, 1989.

PATIENT 13

A 52-year-old woman with a painful bump on her foot

A 52-year-old woman presents with a painful bump on the dorsomedial aspect of her right foot. It has been present for many years and has grown slightly during this time, but has never been painful. It is now especially uncomfortable in tight shoe gear. There has been no trauma to the foot that could have led to development of the bump. The patient has changed shoe gear in an attempt to accommodate the lesion. She denies the presence of other soft-tissue masses elsewhere on her body. There is no significant past medical history; the patient is not taking any medications; and she has no known drug allergies. Review of systems is negative for fever/chills/night sweats, recent weight loss, cough and shortness of breath, nausea/vomiting, and diarrhea or constipation.

Physical Examination: Pedal pulses: bilateral palpable. Vascular: capillary refill time normal. Skin: no edema, normal temperature. Palpation: firm and freely movable mass, approximately 3 cm × 1 cm, on dorsomedial aspect of right foot; location just lateral to tibialis anterior tendon (not within tendon). Aspiration: no fluid within mass.

Laboratory Findings: Radiograph (right foot): soft-tissue swelling over dorsomedial aspect; cortex of first metatarsal and medial cuneiform intact, with no periosteal reaction or invasion; no ossification within lesion.

Question: Considering the histologic findings, what is your diagnosis?

Diagnosis: Benign fibrous histiocytoma

Discussion: This is a common soft-tissue lesion that has also been referred to as a dermatofibroma or sclerosing hemangioma. It is most commonly found on the lower extremity and has a higher incidence in women. It usually comes about after some type of innocuous trauma; some have proposed that an insect bite is causative. The lesion generally is a firm papule or nodule varying in size from 3 to 10 cm. The color is quite variable.

A somewhat pathognomonic sign of a dermatofibroma is the so-called **dimple sign.** When the lesion is squeezed between the forefinger and thumb, a characteristic dimple is produced in the center of the lesion. This dimple is caused by the tethering of the lesion to the overlying epidermis.

Generally, the lesion causes no symptoms that would require its excision, and it frequently regresses in size. In those rare cases when pain is persistent, the lesion can be excised.

The present patient underwent an excisional biopsy. The lesion was excised in toto and sent to pathology, where it was revealed to be a fibrous histiocytoma. This lesion's large size required a skin flap closure after excision, due to the redundant skin that remained following its removal.

Clinical Pearls

1. Histiocytomas can be confused with melanomas because of the change in skin color.
2. Histiocytomas are a variety of dermatofibromas, which are rarely malignant.
3. The treatment is simple excision.

REFERENCES
1. McGlamry ED, et al : Comprehensive Textbook of Foot Surgery, 2nd ed. Baltimore, Williams & Wilkins, 1992.
2. Pearson A, Wolford R: Management of Skin Trauma. Prim Care 27(2): 2000.
3. Potter GK, Ward KA: Tumors. In McGlamry ED, Banks AS, Downey MS (eds): Comprehensive Textbook of Foot Surgery, 2nd ed. Baltimore, Williams & Wilkins, Baltimore, 1992.

PATIENT 14

A 71-year-old man with an itchy, scaly rash on his upper and lower extremities and a lesion on his right foot

A 71-year-old man with a past medical history significant for chronic lymphagenous lymphoma presents with a dry, scaly, red rash on both his upper and lower extremities, face and trunk. The patient recalls the rash beginning 3 years ago, but then disappearing at the end of the summer. It returned 1 year ago.

Physical Examination: Vital signs: normal. General: no distress. HEENT: coarsening of facial features. Cardiac: regular rate, no murmurs. Chest: clear breath sounds. Abdomen: soft, nontender; red, raised, scaly plaques. Extremities: more plaques; bullous lesion at right medial arch. Neurological: intact; no focal deficits.

Laboratory Findings: WBC 12,800/μl (normal 5000–10,000). Buffy coat (abnormal circulating T-cells). Serum chemistry: increased LDH isoenzymes 1,2,3. Chest x-ray: hilar lymphadenopathy. Positive for human T-lymphotropic virus (-1).

Question: What syndrome explains this patient's signs and symptoms?

Diagnosis: Mycosis fungoides (cutaneous T-cell lymphoma [CTCL])

Discussion: Mycosis fungoides or CTCL is a malignancy of CD4 helper T-cells that usually first manifests in the skin. The neoplastic process involves the entire lymphoreticular system, and the lymph nodes and internal organs become involved in the course of the disease. Epidemiologically, this disorder has a 2:1 male to female ratio, and the age range is 5–70 years with typical onset in the 6th or 7th decade of life. The causative agent is believed to be the human T-lymphotropic virus (HTLV), which often is not easily detected initially.

The patient typically reports onset of large, pruritic, red, and scaly plaques perhaps as recently as 1 month, but also as long as several years, ago. These plaques, which are round or arciform-shaped, can be randomly distributed over the entire body. Peripheral lymphadenopathy is often present, and many times the patient has preceding diagnoses such as psoriasis, contact dermatitis, and nummular dermatitis. Chest x-ray reveals a hilar lymphadenopathy, and hematologic exam shows eosinophilia, T-cells, and increased WBC (20,000 ml). Serum chemistry demonstrates increased lactate dehydrogenase isoenzymes 1,2,3.

CT scans are helpful with more advanced stages of the disease and may aid in discovering retroperitoneal nodes in patients with extensive skin involvement, lymphadenopathy, or tumors of the skin. Diagnosis in the early stages is often problematic, and histologic confirmation may not be possible for years despite repeated biopsies.

Dermatopathology of this disorder includes: (1) mycosis cells, which are T-cells with hyperchromatic, irregular-shaped nuclei, in the epidermis and dermis skin layers; (2) microabscesses in the epidermis with mycosis cells; and (3) band-like and patchy infiltrate in the upper dermis extending into skin appendages. Monoclonal antibody techniques are useful, as mycosis cells are activated CD4 T-helper cells.

The course and prognosis of the disease is unpredictable, but the survival rate generally decreases if tumors and lymphadenopathy are present and more than 10% of the skin surface is involved.

Treatment for mycosis fungoides is stage-dependent. In the pre-CTCL stage, with an established histologic diagnosis, PUVA photochemotherapy is the most effective treatment. In the histologically proven plaque stage without lymphademopathy, PUVA photochemotherapy is also the method of choice. For the extensive plaque stage with multiple tumors or in the presence of lymphodenopathy or abnormal circulating T-cells, electron beam plus chemotherapy is probably the best current combination.

Clinical Pearls

1. Biopsy with histologic evaluation may or may not give the diagnosis of cutaneous T-cell lymphoma initially.

2. Look for hilar lymphademopathy on chest x-ray.

3. On physical exam, look for peripheral lymphadenopathy with red, raised, round to arciform-shaped, pruritic plaques.

4. Histologic exam will reveal mycosis cells (T-cells with hyperchromatic, irregularly shaped nuclei).

REFERENCES
1. Fitzpatric T: Color Atlas and Synopsis of Clinical Dermatology, 3rd ed. New York, McGraw-Hill, 1997.
2. Glusac E, et al: Cutaneous T-cell lymphoma. Dermatol Clin 17(3), 1999.

PATIENT 15

A 51-year-old man with chronic diabetic foot ulcerations

A 51-year-old man presents with a 3-month history of ulceration at the 2nd submetatarsal. The patient recalls that after wearing an old pair of shoes, a callus formed and progressively increased to an ulcer. The patient saw his primary care physician, who then referred him to the wound care center. Past medical history is significant for diabetes mellitus.

Physical Examination: Vital signs: normal. General: no distress. HEENT: NCAT. Cardiac: regular rate without murmurs. Chest: clear breath sounds. Abdomen: soft and nontender. Extremities: small, probing ulceration of 2nd submetatarsal, with yellow, foul-smelling drainage, mostly fibrous base, and hyperkeratotic rim; palpable pedal pulses bilaterally; decreased protective sensation to Semmes-Weinstein 5.07 monofilament from toes to midfoot.

Laboratory Findings: WBC 14,200/μl. Radiographs of right foot (see figure): increased sclerosis and lysis of 1st and 2nd metatarsal heads, with bony erosions and loss of architecture; probing soft tissue ulcer below 2nd metatarsal head on lateral view; no soft tissue emphysema evident.

Question: What are some treatment options for this patient?

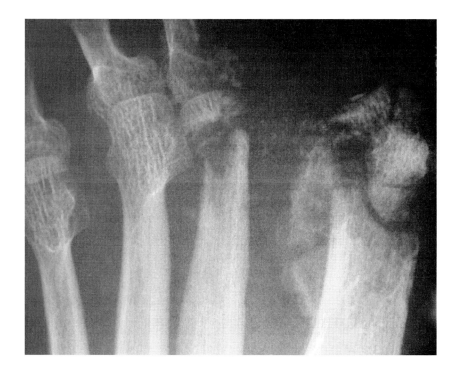

Diagnosis: Osteomyelitis of the 2nd metatarsal

Discussion: Osteomyelitis of the diabetic foot is often a challenge to treat and eradicate, because peripheral vascular disease is usually coexisting. With compromised circulation, delivery of systemic antibiotics (ABX) to the afffected area may be null. Therefore, alternative methods of delivery must be employed. In 1970, Buchholz and Engelbrecht first described the use of ABX-impregnated cement for the treatment of infected total hip arthroplasties. This technique was modified by Calhoun et al in 1994 to the form of ABX polymethylmethacrylate (PMMA) beads on surgical wire for the treatment of osteomyelitis in the ischemic foot.

Commercially prepared ABX-impregnated PMMA beads are not available in the U.S. mainly because of the lack of completed clinical trials. However, most surgeons prepare their own ABX-impregnated beads intraoperatively. PMMA is a compound used to cement the components in place during arthoplasty surgery. The ABX beads are fabricated by implanting antibiotic powder into PMMA cement at a ratio of 5:1. Typically, PMMA cement is distributed in 40s packets, and to avoid excess waste, half of the package can be mixed with the appropriate ratio of ABX. Too much ABX prevents the beads from hardening, whereas too little ABX limits the effectiveness of the beads.

Choice of ABX depends upon the type of microbial infection suspected. Aminoglycosides such as gentamicin, vancomycin, and tobramycin are the most widely used, due to the extensive research available on these ABX, low incidence of reaction, broad spectrum of activity, and heat stability. PMMA cement hardens via an exothermic reaction; therefore, the ABX must be heat stable and water soluble. When possible, choice of ABX-impregnated beads should be directed per culture and sensitivity. Other ABX choices include cefazolin, ticarcillin, pipercillin and doxycycline.

Antibiotic beads are fabricated intraoperatively by mixing pharmaceutical-grade, powdered antibiotic and liquid methlymethacrylate into a putty-like consistency. Next, while the PMMA mixture is still soft, small beads or pellets approximately 3–7 mm in diameter are rolled. The beads are then placed on stainless-steel surgical wire or nonabsorbable suture (no. 10–15). The beads harden in roughly 5–10 minutes via an exothermic reaction—therefore, the surgeon must work efficiently. Following debridement and excision of all devitalized soft tissue and bone, the string of beads is placed loosely into the void of the wound, either completely buried or left with one bead exposed (see figure). The skin is then closed primarily.

Typically the string of beads is left in for 2 weeks. However, if the need exists to fill a dead space or if risk of a second procedure to remove the beads is not advisable, the beads can remain permanently without causing adverse effects. Two weeks is the period within which the beads can be removed with minimal granulation tissue overgrowth. Note that the beads can be removed in toto, or inched out one at a time as the granulation tissue fills the wound. If the wound cannot be primarily closed, an occlusive film dressing can be employed to form an ABX bead pouch.

The benefit of this procedure is the ability to achieve high levels of ABX concentration at a local site while avoiding systemic toxicity. The closed space is a requirement to obtain a high, local concentration of the ABX. The ABX is then released into the wound by diffusion. Elution of the ABX is greatest within the first 48 hours and then tapers down over the next couple of months. Detectable levels of ABX have been recorded in beads implanted over 4 years.

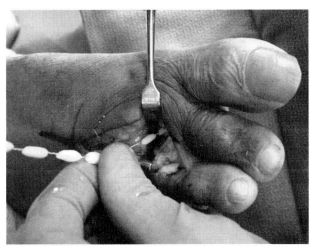

Small-sized beads (3–7 mm diameter) are ideal because increased surface area allows a large percentage of ABX to be released at a quicker rate. ABX-impregnated PMMA beads avoid adverse side effects and systemic toxicity. They are especially useful when managing patients in whom achieving therapeutic tissue levels of ABX in the foot is difficult, such as those with diabetes mellitus or infrapopliteal occlusive artery.

In the present patient, resection, biopsy, and insertion of antibiotic-impregnated beads were used to eradicate this osteomyelitic process.

Clinical Pearls

1. Use heat-stable, powdered ABX and liquid PMMA cement to prepare antibiotic beads. Mix ABX with cement 5:1 respectively.

2. Make small-diameter beads and use stainless-steel surgical wire or nonabsorbable suture.

3. Close the wound primarily, or use occlusive film dressing over it.

4. Beads can remain permanently without adverse effects, or can be removed.

REFERENCES

1. Henry SL: ABX-impregnated beads. Part 1. Ortho Rev 20(3): 242–247, 1991
2. Henry SL: Local ABX treatment for management of orthotic infections. Clin Pharmokinetics 29(1): 36–45, 1995,
3. Roeder B, et al: Antibiotic beads in the treatment of DM pedal osteomyelitis. J Foot Ankle Surg 39(2):124–130, 2000.

PATIENT 16

A 74-year-old man with nontraumatic heel pain

A 74-year-old man presents with a 3-week history of right heel pain. He relates receiving a steroid injection from his primary care physician 2 weeks ago, which did offer some relief. The patient describes severe pain over the last couple of days, increased with activity and when he wears his dress shoes. He has obtained only minimal relief from anti-inflammatories. He denies any trauma to the area.

Physical Examination: Vital signs: stable. HEENT: normal. Cardiac: regular rate and rhythm. Chest: clear. Abdomen: benign. Skin: normal. Neurological: motor and sensory intact. Lower extremity: palpable pedal pulses; mild tenderness with palpation of plantar medial tubercle of right heel, negative discomfort along plantar fascia, significant pain with medial and lateral compression of calcaneus, no tenderness noted to insertion of Achilles tendon, negative Tinel's sign, no evidence of erythema, ecchymosis, or edema.

Laboratory Findings: CBC: normal. Uric acid: 5 mg/dl. Rheumatoid factor: negative. Radiographs: small plantar calcaneal spur of right foot; negative cortical or bony disruption. Tc99 bone scan (see figure): intensely increased activity on all three phases within the right heel.

Questions: What is the cause of this patient's heel pain? Describe the recommended treatment.

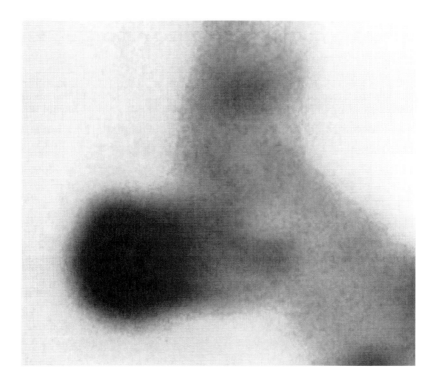

Diagnosis: Stress fracture right calcaneus

Discussion: Stress fractures of the foot are mainly localized to the 2nd metatarsal and calcaneus. The mechanism of injury, which is common to all stress fractures, is excessive repetitive force that causes fatigue and eventually fracture. The body responds to this repetitive stress by laying down new bone trabeculations along the lines of increased stress, which can take up to 2 weeks. If the repetitive force continues during this process, the body does not have a chance to lay down new trabeculae, and failure ensues. The primarily cancellous calcaneus reacts with a compression-type fracture usually perpendicular to the trabeculations at the junction of the body and tuberosity. This does not become apparent on radiographs until 2 weeks from date of injury.

Consider the diagnosis of stress fracture in any patient that presents with heel pain. Patients usually present with point tenderness to the plantar calcaneus, and describe pain that increases throughout the day and is often aggravated by lack of cushioning in shoe gear. Occasionally, patients relate a recent history of beginning a running routine or weight gain. A variety of metabolic diseases including osteomalacia, osteogenesis imperfecta, hyperparathyroidism, scurvy, Paget's disease, fibrous dysplasia, and even rheumatoid arthritis predispose a patient to develop stress fractures.

Findings are often similar to plantar fasciitis, but patients do not complain of post static dyskinesia—rather, pain increases with continued activity. The classic clinical finding is severe pain with lateral compression of the calcaneus and minimal tenderness of the plantar medial tubercle.

Plain radiographs appear normal at the onset of symptoms. The most useful diagnostic modality is a three-phase Tc99 bone scan, which shows focal uptake within the calcaneus as early as 2 days following fracture. An MRI may also be helpful, showing signs of marrow edema (decreased signal intensity on T1-weighted image).

The earlier the patient presents for treatment, the better he or she responds. An injection for plantar fasciitis should be avoided if there is any suspicion of stress fracture due to delayed healing or avascular necrosis of the calcaneus. If diagnosed early enough, a stress reaction may be all that is present. These patients respond quickly to 1–2 weeks of nonweight-bearing with crutches, soft cast, and gradual return to activity. Once a definitive fatigue fracture has been diagnosed, ample time must be given to allow for complete healing. Ideally, a short leg cast and removal of weight-bearing until the fracture is nontender (usually 4–6 weeks) is the treatment of choice. A cam walker and an ACE bandage may be used for immobilization if the patient is not able to maintain non-weight bearing.

The present patient was placed in a below-knee cast for a total of 6 weeks. He was instructed to remain non-weight bearing for this time with the aid of a rolling walker. After the cast was removed, the patient slowly increased physical activity. He remained asymptomatic and was able to return to normal daily activities.

Clinical Pearls

1. A calcaneal stress fracture may present similarly to plantar faciitis, but the patient is significantly more tender on lateral compression.

2. If there is any suspicion of fracture, a corticosteroid injection should be avoided.

3. Obtain a bone scan or MRI if the patient states that pain increases throughout the day, and there is point tenderness and pain with compression of the calcaneus.

4. A three-phase Tc99 bone scan shows increased uptake in all three phases with a positive stress fracture.

5. Treatment of calcaneal stress fractures includes immobilization with a short leg cast and nonweight-bearing for at least 4–6 weeks.

REFERENCE

Brighton CT: Principles of fracture healing. Instr Course Lect 33:60, 1984.

PATIENT 17

A 52-year-old man with an 8-month history of a foot ulcer

A 52-year-old man is admitted to the hospital because of an ulcer under the 2nd metatarsal head of the right foot. The ulcer has been present for approximately 8 months. It is approximately 10 mm in depth with 5 mm of undermining, and the wound is 7 × 9 mm. The patient received weekly treatments in a wound-care facility. Treatment consisted of a variety of wound-care products, sharp debridement, and accommodative and offloading shoes. All of these measures were unsuccessful in healing the ulcer.

He is a type 2 diabetic with a 30-year history of diabetes. History includes alcohol abuse and a 3-pack-a-day smoking addiction. He is allergic to penicillin. Current medications include glyburide, 2.5 mg/day; ciprofloxacin, 750 mg by mouth, twice daily; clindamycin, 300 mg by mouth, every 6 hours.

Physical Examination: General: well-developed, well-nourished, in no distress. Temperature 98.8° F, pulse 88, respirations 18, blood pressure 110/70 in the supine position. Skin: ulcer under 2nd metatarsal head of right foot; bone exposed; no signs of cellulitis and minimal serous drainage. Musculoskeletal: strength 5/5 in all extremities; deep tendon reflexes: normal. Neurological: total sensory loss of right foot when tested with a 5.07 Semmes-Weinstein monofilament.

Laboratory Findings: WBC 4900/μl, glucose 180 mg/dl, ESR 52 mm/hr, hemoglobin 13.1 g/dl, hct 37.6%. *Imaging:* Radiographs of right foot—loss of distal portion of 2nd metatarsal head; periosteal new bone formation (see figure). Three-phase technetium-99m bone scan—increased uptake in delayed phase of 2nd and 3rd metatarsals; no other uptake noted within foot or ankle. Noninvasive arterial blood flow studies—triphasic wave forms at dorsalis pedis, posterior tibial, and popliteal arteries; pressures of 70 mmHg at second toe and 110 mmHg at transmetatarsal level; ankle-brachial index 0.9.

Questions: Describe your diagnostic impression. How would you proceed?

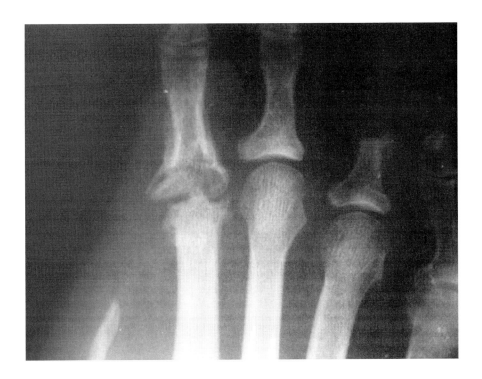

Diagnosis: Osteomyelitis of the 2nd metatarsal

Discussion: Certainly a bone biopsy and culture is the gold standard in the diagnosis of osteomyelitis, giving the absolute information needed for further treatment. In the present patient, the pathology report revealed multiple areas of plasma cells, osteonecrosis, and inflammatory responses consistent with osteomyelitis. The demineralization process confirmed the presence of osteomyelitis microscopically. The microbiology results of the bone specimen revealed *Staphylococcus aureus,* which was methicillin-resistant.

The patient underwent a proximal transmetatarsal amputation and received a 6-week course of IV vancomycin through a Hickman. He was kept offloaded during the entire postoperative course, and upon complete closure of the wound site, he was fitted with a molded shoe and toe filler.

This form of osteomyelitis tends to be chronic. The patient did not fit the systemic illness pattern, but rather had a localized disease process. Persistent drainage may be the only finding from a small sinus tract. All too often, the patient ignores this finding, or the practitioner ignores the potential danger. Rarely does the patient feel pain or even see redness until the area becomes superficially infected. It is not until the radiographs reveal the typical findings of thickened, irregular-shaped sclerotic bone with areas of radiolucency and areas of periostium elevation that the alarm is sounded.

A radical approach is critical, as local antibiotic or IV therapy is usually unsuccessful. Inadequate treatment leaves a low-grade infection that persists and may explode into an infective process—which again is treated inappropriately. In the patient described here, the 2nd metatarsal head is in a destructive radiolucent phase; if this follows its chronic nature, a layering of eburnated periostium will develop, resulting in a shortening of the 2nd metatarsal with a shift and transfer of weight to the adjacent metatarsal head. This area will then break open into another ulcer, further complicating this diabetic patient's ambulatory status.

Clinical Pearls

1. As important as it is to recognize and diagnose osteomyelitis early, it is more important to isolate the organisms creating the infection early in the process.

2. Bone cultures via an adjacent site or excision of the bone in question is imperative for a complete diagnosis.

3. In a diabetic patient, if bone is exposed for any period of time, osteomyelitis should be at the top of your differential diagnosis list.

REFERENCES

1. McGlamry E, Banks A, Downey M: Comprehensive Textbook of Foot Surgery, 2nd ed. Baltimore, MD, Williams & Wilkins, 1992.
2. McKittrick LS, McKittrick JB, Risley TS: Transmetatarsal amputations for infection or gangrene in patients with diabetes mellitus. Ann Surg 130: 826, 1949.

PATIENT 18

A 13-year-old girl with lateral foot pain

The patient presents with complaints of left foot pain of approximately 2-year duration. There is no specific history of a traumatic event. The pain is primarily at the lateral aspect of the foot, is worse at the end of the day, and is somewhat relieved by rest. The child relates that over the past 3 months the pain has increased, and it not relieved by NSAIDs. She is unable to participate in school sports and cannot walk for any long distances.

Physical Examination: General: no swelling of left foot; tender at anterolateral aspect. Musculoskeletal: exquisite pain on ankle plantarflexion; subtalar motion limited; eversion present; peroneal tendons not in spasm; no lateral leg pain; midtarsal joint ROM unattainable. Gait analysis: gastrocnemius equinus, demonstrated by limitation of dorsiflexion at ankle when leg is extended on thigh (increased dorsiflexion when leg is flexed on thigh); longitudinal medial arch decreased with abduction of forefoot.

Laboratory Findings: Radiographs: AP and lateral—beaking of talus and narrowing of subtalar joint; "anteater sign." Medial oblique—calcaneonavicular bony bridge. Harris-Beathe—middle and posterior facets of subtalar joints parallel to one another. CT scan (see figure): bony bridge between calcaneus and navicular, with no changes in subtalar joints.

Questions: What type of coalition is present? What would be an acceptable conservative course of treatment?

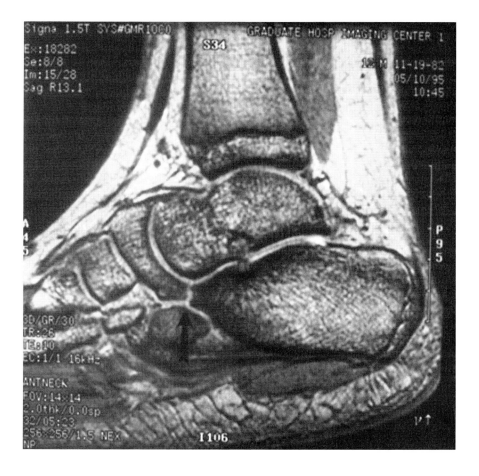

Diagnosis: Calcaneonavicular coalition and secondary gastrocnemius equinus

Discussion: In young children, the most common site for fibrocartilaginous unions is the posterior region of the subtalar joint. Mobilization of the coalesced joint, rather than a fusion, is common practice in the therapy of this disorder. The release of the fibrous tissue can restore motion to the rearfoot. Only when the foot matures (16–18 years of age) does one consider any type of single or multiple joint fusions. Conservative treatment usually fails in the treatment of calcaneonavicular (C-N) bridges. Success is reported when resecting this bridge in the young, active child. Subtalar fusion is not necessary even in the presence of talar beaking in a child with calcaneonavicular coalition.

However, in the adult, the prognosis is worse if talar beaking is present. Simple resection of the C-N bar in the adult and replacement with wax or silicone, or interposing the belly of the extensor digitorum brevis, does not guarantee mobilization. The young child is more active and it is possible that this explains the higher success rate of resection in children.

The difficulty and the usual complication that arises with the young child and their complaint of pain in the rearfoot is misdiagnosis and inappropriate treatment. Without proper visualization of the rearfoot, you cannot treat this condition. CT has certainly helped in the diagnosis of osseous or narrow coalitions, but with the aid of MRI you can isolate the exact position, thickness, and length of the fibrous bond in any of the joints. When the subtalar joint is restricted and the midtarsal joint loses its gliding motion, the talus starts to override the navicular and talar beaking results.

When the coalition is present in a child's early developing stages, the adjacent joint changes as well. Besides the future arthritic changes and adaptive changes (lipping and jamming of joints), another phenomenon occurs: a ball and socket ankle develops as a compensatory response to the restricted motion of the subtalar joint. The tibial plafond becomes concave, and the dome appears to be convex and ball-shaped; the joint now accepts full ROM in dorsiflexion, plantarflexion, inversion, and eversion. Ankle stability is at risk, however, since the foot is in a valgus position. (Note: After fusion, this is the position to strive for—the instability is not pronounced.) If the pain is extreme, cast the foot in slight pronation—do not invert. A period of immobilization (3–6 weeks) may be attempted using this short leg walking cast. Rest, ice, and anti-inflammatories may have a positive effect.

In the aging child and the child who develops the coalition late, the result will not be the ball and socket ankle but an ankle with degenerative joint changes. In this situation, a pantalar fusion is required. As with many childhood conditions, early recognition reduces the need for radical, complication-prone procedures. The first course of treatment is by conservative means. A sport orthotic would be well tolerated and allow the foot to pronate slightly. Omit forefoot posting so as not to drive the first ray higher, affecting the midtarsal joint. Do not post the foot in rearfoot varus, as this will allow too much motion to bring the forefoot down. If the midtarsal motion is increased, pain will be increased. Stabilize the heel to decrease the stresses across a stiff subtalar joint. When subtalar joint motion is restricted and the midtarsal joint losses its gliding motion, the talus starts to override the navicular, and talar beaking results.

When all conservative steps fail, consider surgery. Significant relief can be obtained by resection of the coalition. Place a layer of material in the calcaneonavicular space to avoid a recurrence. Resect the bar, and interpose the extensor digitorum brevis.

The present patient failed all conservative measures. She underwent surgical resection of the calcaneonavicular coalition, with interposition of the extensor digitorum brevis muscle. A gastrocnemius lengthening was also performed. A short leg cast was applied postoperatively for a period of 6 weeks. After removal of the cast the patient was placed in custom-molded orthoses. She now enjoys an active childhood and participates in several school sports.

Clinical Pearls

1. Clinical diagnosis is quite important. If a limitation of midtarsal joint motion is noted in light of an acceptable amount of rearfoot motion, then strongly consider calcaneonavicular coalition.

2. After clinical impression, the medial oblique radiograph is key. It allows parallel observation of the joint and easy identification of signs.

3. If in doubt, an MRI will nicely demonstrate fibrous and osseous unions.

4. The CT is most useful when the child is older and an osseous union is suspected over a fibrous.

5. If a secondary gastrocnemius equinus develops because of the abducted position, consider a heel-raised orthotic. If the equinus is significant, perhaps lengthen the tendon at the time of resection.

REFERENCES

1. Gonzalez P, Jayakumar S: Calcaneonavicular coalition treated by resection and interposition of the extensor digitorum brevis muscle. J Bone Joint Surg 72A:71–77, 1990.
2. Herzenberg JE, Gldner JL, Martinez S, Silverman PM: Computerized tomography of talocalcaneal tarsal coalition. Foot Ankle 6(6):273–288, 1986.
3. Mosier KM, Asher M: Tarsal coalitions and peroneal spastic flat foot. J Bone Joint Surg 66A:976–984, 1984.

PATIENT 19

A 15-year-old girl with pain in her second toe

A 15-year-old girl presents with left foot pain near the second toe. The pain has been present for 1 year. She has no history of trauma, and describes the pain as a constant, dull ache that has been getting progressively worse. She also reveals that the pain increases when she wears high-heeled shoes.

Physical Examination: Musculoskeletal: exquisite tenderness at metatarsal with flexion and extension of left second toe; tenderness on palpation over dorsum of 2nd metatarsophalangeal joint; extreme pain on forcible compression of phalanx base against 2nd metatarsal head. Gait analysis: patient places majority of her weight on lateral aspect; forefoot inverted.

Laboratory Findings: Radiographs: AP view (see figure)—flattening of metatarsal head and joint space widening with a central depression; lateral view—cleft in dorsal head/neck region with slight beaking, and small osteophytic fragment near joint level.

Questions: What is your first impression? What are your surgical options?

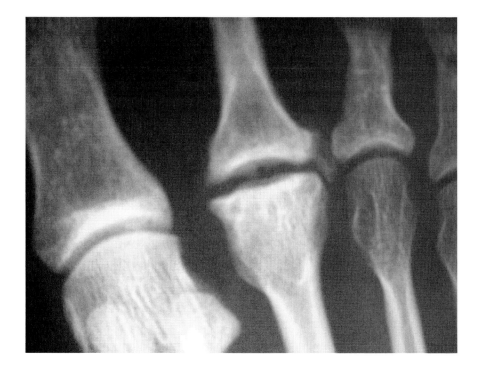

Diagnosis: Freiberg's infraction

Discussion: A plausible theory for the failure of this articular epiphysis to heal is constant compression. Delayed union and poor endochondral ossification are the result. Constant trauma to an immature epiphysis changes the mechanical efforts exerted by the joint. The normal rotation about the articular surface ceases and is replaced by direct compression. If left unchecked over the years, the joint will become rigid, painful, and osteoarthritic.

Radiographically, the most obvious finding is widening of the joint space. This widening occurs by the sixth week after symptom onset. With progression of the condition, the density of the subchondral bone increases, and the metatarsal head flattens. In the advanced stage in the older child, the ischemic epiphyseal bone and articular cartilage weaken and collapse. The collapsed bone creates fracturing within the joint, and loose bodies appear, with resultant pain. It is not unusual to see these fragments in the dorsal aspect of the joint space.

The least traumatic and certainly the most ambulatory surgery entails removal of the fragment. Resecting the dorsal aspect of the metatarsal head allows for increased dorsal range of motion. Resection of the proximal phalanx base decompresses the metatarsal head and usually reduces the symptoms. In time, however, weight as well as pressure on the surrounding metatarsal heads will increase, creating a transfer lesion.

Perforating the subchondral surface by drilling is an option if considered early in the development of Freiberg's. Penetration through the metatarsal head, epiphysis, and metatarsal shaft causes increased blood to be delivered to the distal aspect. It may be advisable to consider an osteotomy to realign the metatarsal head. This would eliminate the direct compression on the head from the plantar weight-bearing surface. In addition, rotating the head effects a decrease in the retrograde force from the phalanx.

Joint destructive procedures should be avoided in children; however, if the pain is significant, and the damage to the articular portion is extensive, you may be led to resect the metatarsophalangeal joint completely or partially. Implants are not contraindicated. Pain with this deformity is exhausting to the child *and* to the parents; if all else has failed, then this radical approach is recommended.

In the present patient, the treatment was radical due to the extensive damage to the articular surface.

Clinical Pearls

1. Early recognition of Freiberg's infraction is paramount. Offloading the joint with decompression has proved successful.

2. An orthotic constructed to maintain a forefoot varus as well as forefoot extension, with a cut-out to allow the 2nd metatarsal to drop, decreases jamming of the second toe.

3. Consider an early dorsiflexory osteotomy on the neck of the metatarsal to increase dorsiflexion. This is similar to a Waterman procedure, and will increase motion.

REFERENCES

1. Binek R, et al: Freiberg's disease complicating unrelated trauma. Orthopedics 11:5:753–757, 1988.
2. Canale S, Beaty J: Operative Pediatric Orthopedics, 2nd ed. St. Louis, MO, Mosby, 1995.
3. Drennan J: The Child's Foot and Ankle. New York, Raven Press, 1992.
4. Helal B, Gibb P: Freiberg's disease. Foot Ankle 8:94–102, 1987.
5. Kinnard P, Lirette R: Dorsiflexion osteotomy in Freiberg's disease. Foot Ankle 9:226–231, 1989.
6. Meehan P: Lovell and Winter's Pediatric Orthopaedics, 3rd ed. Philadelphia, Lippincott, 1990.
7. Sproul J, et al: Surgical treatment of Freiberg's infraction in athletes. Am J Sports Med 21(3): 381–384, 1993.

PATIENT 20

A 13-year-old girl with a painful foot

A 13-year-old girl has been complaining of pain in her left foot for 3 months. Conservative home remedies did not provide any significant relief. Her chief complaint is acute pain localized within the sinus tarsi and pain corresponding to the course of the peroneal tendons along the lateral aspect of her left foot. The left foot is more symptomatic than right. Playing sports especially aggravates the problem. She experiences greatest pain when walking barefoot. The patient's past medical history is unremarkable. Family history includes maternal talonavicular synostosis and symptomatic subtalar coalition.

Physical Examination: Pedal pulses: steady and palpable. Skin: normal. Neurologic: normal. General: rearfoot valgus bilaterally, with forefoot perpendicular to rearfoot; gastrocnemius equinus bilaterally; mild hallux abducto valgus with valgus rotation of interphalangeal joint and contracted digits two through five bilaterally. Musculoskeletal: hip, knee, and ankle joint ROM normal; subtalar and midtarsal joint ROM restricted bilaterally; muscle strength normal and symmetrical. Gait analysis: antalgic apropulsive cycle.

Laboratory Findings: Radiographs: talonavicular synostosis and subtalar coalition; talar beaking; narrowing of posterior talocalcaneal space; rounding of lateral process of talus; middle subtalar joint obliteration on lateral view; asymmetry of anterior facet of subtalar joint in lateral oblique; halo effect (continuous sclerotic rim around sustentaculum tali); irregular and hazy cortical surface surrounding coalition; no distinct cortical margins; secondary degenerative joint disease and ball-and-socket ankle (BASA) joint (see figure).

Course: Initially she was given a peroneal nerve block with 2% lidocaine, which relieved a peroneal spasm. Subsequently a sinus tarsi injection was administered with 2% lidocaine, methylprednisolone 40 mg/ml, and dexamethasone 4 mg/ml, and a Unna boot was applied. The patient was instructed to walk with crutches, nonweight-bearing. After 3 months of conservative therapy, she is still experiencing significant pain while walking.

Question: Why is the patient still experiencing pain after 3 months of conservative therapy?

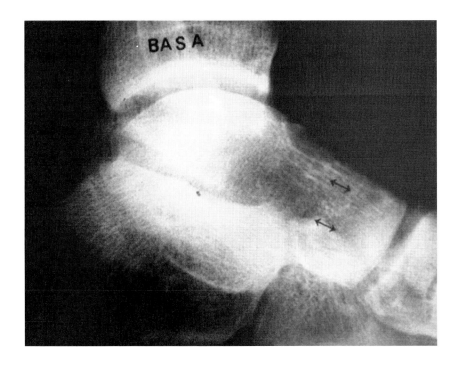

Diagnosis: Talonavicular coalition and subtalar coalition

Discussion: Most of the present patient's discomfort was relieved by a limitation of motion. The most common presentation of talonavicular synostosis is local tenderness over the coalition site, enhanced by activity and relieved by immobilization or rest. However, the pain is referred to a proximal joint. In this case it was the subtalar joint. Pain is usually deep within the sinus tarsi, and a restriction of subtalar joint and midtarsal joint range of motion is characteristic.

Peroneal spasm may be present, but not necessarily. Peroneal spasm is frequently found in medial talocalcaneal coalitions, the most common tarsal coalition, in which there is a restriction of motion on the medial aspect of the joint, but not laterally. This ultimately leads to a calcaneovalgus deformity, with a decrease in the medial longitudinal arch and abduction of the forefoot.

With most coalitions, motion is transferred to the adjacent joint. In this patient, the motion was picked up by the ankle. Since this was an early-onset synostosis, the talar dome began rounding to create a ball-and-socket ankle. This development increased inversion and eversion. The solution to the patient's persistent pain was a deep-seated heel seat to prevent the increased frontal plane motion of the ankle.

Clinical Pearls

1. Early identification of a synostosis with protection of the proximal joints decreases the chance of joint arthritis as the child grows.

2. In early fusing of joints, the restriction of motion only increases proximal joint motion. Always evaluate the ankle for the potential development of a ball-and-socket joint (limitation of motion distally, with a resultant increase motion proximally).

REFERENCES

1. Cowell HR, Elener V: Rigid painful flatfoot secondary to tarsal coalition. Clin Orthop 177:54, 1983.
2. Downey MS: Tarsal coalition. In Comprehensive Textbook of Foot Surgery. Vol 1. Baltimore, Williams & Wilkins, 1992, pp 898–930.
3. Jacobs AM, Sollecito V, Oloff LM, Klein N: Tarsal coalitions: An instructional review. J Foot Surg 20(4), 1981.

PATIENT 21

A 14-year-old boy with severe foot pain causing him to crawl

The patient usually is a very active child. Until recently, he played sports all year round. Over the past 3 months he has been complaining of increasing pain over the lateral aspect of his right foot. He can no longer play any sport. When he has been walking for a long period the pain is so intense that he begins to crawl. Upon questioning, he points directly to the area of the sinus tarsi. The use of ice and a nonsteroidal anti-inflammatory drug has offered him some relief. An over-the-counter insert he purchased also has somewhat mitigated the pain.

Physical Examination: General: overall health very good. Lower extremity: limitation of mid-tarsal and subtalar motion; moderate swelling of right foot compared to left. Neurovascular: normal. Gait analysis: stance—right foot abducted with loss of medial longitudinal arch and everted heel to ground position; gait—early heel-off with marked abduction of foot to leg.

Laboratory Findings: Radiographs (see figures): lateral view—elongated anterosuperior process of calcaneus, known as anteater sign; medial oblique view—calcaneus and navicular in close proximity; bones appear flattened with irregular, indistinct cortical surfaces. MRI: changed signals on the T2-weighted image.

Question: What is the likelihood that this deformity will eventually require surgical intervention?

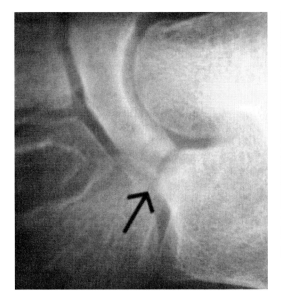
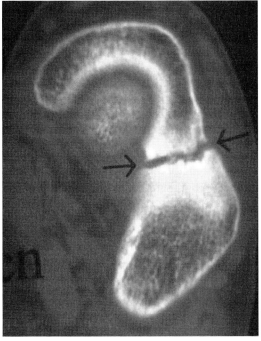

Answer: Thirty-five percent of soft tissue calcaneonavicular coalitions eventually require surgery.

Discussion: Pain is a common finding in this condition, and is usually insidious in onset following some recent activity or trauma. Limitation of subtalar and midtarsal joint motion is an obvious clinical finding. The subtalar joint is usually limited in the direction of inversion, with greater limitation if peroneal muscle spasm is present. Patients may present with a valgus deformity due to intense tonic peroneus brevis spasm, which is simply a reflex mechanism to limit painful inversion. Inversion and eversion of the midtarsal joint induce pain. With time, the valgus deformity becomes more rigid. There are, however, several reported cases of spasticity of muscles other than the peroneus brevis and of a varus position of the heel in patients with calcaneonavicular coalitions.

Pain is usually isolated to the midtarsal joint region, and the child points directly to the area of the sinus tarsi. With limitation of midtarsal and subtalar joints, the foot begins to compensate in the direction of abduction and eversion. The peroneals shorten up due to this compensated position. Any attempt to invert or plantarflex the foot creates extreme pain. Unfortunately, a peroneal spastic flatfoot often is diagnosed inappropriately.

Calcaneonavicular coalitions are usually identifiable on the medial oblique view. This coalition typically appears as a 1-cm wide bar bridging the gap normally found between the calcaneus and navicular. A "pseudocoalition" due to bony overlap can give the false impression of a calcaneonavicular bar, making it necessary to obtain several medial oblique views at different angles to differentiate between positional artifact and true coalition. In the case of a fibrous or cartilaginous calcaneonavicular coalition, the diagnosis will be more difficult. On the lateral view, an elongated anterosuperior process of the calcaneus, known as the **anteater sign,** may be seen. The calcaneus and navicular are closer than normal on the medial oblique view, and the bones appear flattened with irregular, indistinct cortical surfaces.

MRI virtually eliminates the difficulty in diagnosis of soft tissue, and provides the physician with an advantage when he or she suspects nonosseous coalitions. Although relatively invisible on conventional radiography, fibrous or cartilaginous unions can be confirmed with the use of MRI. Radiographs and CT have not proven reliable in the identification of fibrous tarsal coalitions. MRI accurately and reliably indicates fibrous, cartilaginous, and osseous coalitions of the talocalcaneal and calcaneonavicular joints, and is useful for detecting the presence of coexisting bars. MRI is recommended with suspected tarsal coalitions when radiography and CT are negative.

Early intervention is paramount. Young children that present with talar beaking secondary to compensation respond favorably to resection of the calcaneonavicular soft tissue coalition. When talar beaking is present in the older child or young adult, response is less favorable, and a triple arthrodesis is generally necessary.

Conservative treatment is aimed at restriction of subtalar and midtarsal joint motion to reduce pain. This may be accomplished through the use of shoe modifications, orthoses, padding, or casting. Physical therapy, anti-inflammatory medications, and local steroid injection into the area of the coalition may be used as adjuncts. Although the symptoms may resolve for a time, they may recur in the future, requiring repeated casting or even surgical intervention.

In the present patient, a resection was inevitable, and the child was then maintained in an orthosis to minimize midtarsal motion.

Clinical Pearls

1. Isolate the midtarsal joint by stabilizing the heel with your hand, maintaining a neutral postion. Abduct-dorsiflex the foot and then repeat in a plantarflexory adducted position. Two things happen with a coalition: pain is elicited over the sinus tarsi, and a limitation of motion is noted.

2. MRI is recommend as the best diagnostic aid for a suspected coalition.

REFERENCES
1. Downey MS: Tarsal coalitions: A surgical classification. J Am Podiatr Med Assoc 81:187, 1991.
2. Pachuda NM, Lasday SD, Jay RM: Tarsal coalition: Etiology, diagnosis, and treatment. J Foot Surg 29:474, 1990.
3. Penman MD, Wertheimer SJ: Tarsal coalitions. J Foot Surg 25:1986.

PATIENT 22

An 8-year-old girl with nightly heel pain

A healthy, athletic little girl complains of severe right foot pain at the end of the day and in the middle of the night. Her parents state that she awakes in tears as the entire foot is painful. The pain has been present for over 9 months and has been increasing in severity. It centers around the lower ankle and heel. The family doctor attributed the pain to increased activity and "growing pains." The girl's pediatrician advised the parents to take her to a podiatrist for orthotic devices. The devices afforded her no relief, and she was referred for a second opinion.

The patient's past medical history is uneventful, with no history of trauma. She experiences a decrease in pain when aspirin is administered.

Physical Examination: General: stiffness and guarding around subtalar joint, plus decrease in total ROM; right calf muscle atrophy (thinner than opposite extremity by 1 cm). Musculoskeletal: pain localized to right arch and heel area both medially and laterally; no pain upon posterior compression of calcaneus, nor upon active dorsiflexion of ankle. Skin: no signs of inflammation or edema; vascular supply to foot excellent.

Laboratory Findings: Radiographs (see figure): lateral view—opaque, halo-like area 1 cm in diameter, resting inferior and posterior to the sustentaculum tali; axial view (of calcaneus, directed 0 degrees to superior surface)—similar findings, with halo located approximately 2 cm from lateral wall of the calcaneus. Technetium 99 three-phase bone scan: focal area of increased perfusion in region of right calcaneus; immediate and postinjection images—focal area of increased vascularity in region of mid-right calcaneus; static images—increased activity in this region. CT: density in superior margin of right calcaneus body and nidus lucency in inferior margin.

Questions: What is your differential diagnosis? What is the probable diagnosis?

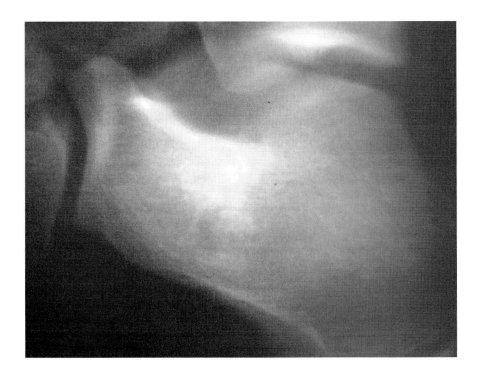

Diagnosis: Osteoid osteoma

Discussion: Osteochondritis, stress fracture, bone islands (enostosis), and Brodies's abscess are suggested by the radiographic modalities. Radiologic studies have proved to be the most valuable diagnostic tool, but the hazy, trabecular pattern of cancellous bone in the young child makes the lesion difficult to locate. There should be a dense, sclerotic rim surrounding the lesion. This, too, is not easily spotted in the very young child with an early developing lesion. The dense rim does not appear until late in the lesion's maturation, when it is being vascularly compressed. If located in the spongy bone layer, the lesion increases in size with referring pain, but does not consolidate a sclerotic rim about the central clear nidus.

Additional studies are recommended in young children presenting with this vague but classic pain, to clearly identify a suspected lesion. Normally, children do not have pain. If pain is present, it must be seriously considered until a firm diagnosis is attained. A lesion may be located in the cortical, cancellous, or subperosteal bone. While all will demonstrate a radiolucent nidus with a sclerotic rim, cancellous and subperiosteal bone lesions are more difficult to diagnose as these features are less pronounced.

In the atypical situation, the nidus is not surrounded by sclerotic bone, which makes it especially difficult to identify within the complex radiological anatomy of the joints. This scenario often leads to misdiagnosis and delayed definitive treatment. Misdiagnoses include post-traumatic synovitis, rheumatoid arthritis, and even hysteria. In many cases, patients undergo unnecessary treatment, such as immobilization with plaster, use of crutches for an extended period of time, joint injections, arthroscopy, and even psychoanalysis.

In the present patient, a CT was obtained, and the osteoid osteoma was identified and surgically resected. A bone graft was placed in the defect. The patient was placed in a below-knee cast for a period of 6 weeks. She went on to heal uneventfully.

Clinical Pearls

1. Pain is the most important clue: *children do not have pain unless there is a disorder present.* When in doubt, check it out. Do not assume hysteria.

2. If there is suspicion of an osteoid osteoma in a young patient with persistent, undiagnosed joint pain, radiological examination, bone scan, and CT should be repeated 1 year after the onset of symptoms, since the initial negative findings may be positive at a later date. Bone scintigraphy and CT aid in the diagnosis. Scintigraphy identifies the affected joint, and CT assists in localizing the precise tumor site.

REFERENCES

1. Huvos AG (ed): Bone Tumors: Diagnosis, Treatment, and Prognosis, 2nd ed. Philadelphia, W.B. Saunders, 1990.
2. Jay RM: Surgical treatment of osteoid osteoma in the adolescent. J Foot Surg 29:495–498, 1990.
3. Kenzora JE: Problems encountered in the diagnosis and treatment of osteoid osteoma of the talus. Foot Ankle 2:172–178, 1981.
4. Resnick D (ed): Diagnosis of Bone and Joint Disorders, 4th ed. Philadelphia, W.B. Saunders, 2001.

PATIENT 23

A 19-month-old girl who is unable to walk

A 19-month-old girl is presented for evaluation of an unstable gait upon ambulation. The parents' primary concern is a falling tendency that has been evident since the child began to walk at 9 months of age.

Physical Examination: Gait analysis: abnormal equinus gait; heels elevated during entire gait cycle; when stationary, heels came down to supporting surface and knees went into genu recurvatum. Neurologic: no delay in development, no deficit; normal for age; equinus congenital, not related to any neuromuscular disease.

Treatment Course: Serial dorsiflexing casts were employed in an attempt to reduce the bilateral equinus and genu recurvatum. The casts were applied in knee extension, from the toes to the proximal thigh, and changed weekly for a 4-week period. Gradually dorsiflexing the foot to decrease the plantarflexion at the ankle reduced the equinus. Following cast removal, reduction of the equinus deformity was maintained. Ankle dorsiflexion was increased to 15 degrees, and the child had a remarkable ability to ambulate.

Approximately 6 weeks after the casts had been removed, the parents observed the child to have some difficulty walking, and within a few weeks she had lost all ability to stand straight. The genu recurvatum returned in compensation of the equinus. The child eventually started leaning so far forward in an effort to maintain balance that she would fall. In a short time she was unable to stand or walk. Casting was reinstated and the possible need for an Achilles tendon–lengthening procedure was discussed.

After 1 month of casting no improvement of the equinus was observed, and casting was discontinued. A consultation with the child's pediatrician revealed that he too had not detected any neurologic abnormalities or developmental delay. With this confusing picture of continual contracture of unknown origin, additional studies were performed prior to the tendo Achilles lengthening.

Laboratory Findings: EMG nerve conduction velocities: no sural nerve sensory response; motor nerve velocities in upper and lower extremities slowed; sensory action potentials diminished in amplitude, with prolonged latency to peak. MRI of brain (T2-weighted images): abnormal increased signal intensity in supratentorial white matter bilaterally, occipital region greater than frontal. Enzyme analysis: arylsulfatase A deficiency.

Question: What is your diagnosis?

Diagnosis: Metachromatic leukodystrophy (MLD)

Discussion: The late infantile form of MLD begins insidiously between the first and second year. It is transmitted as an autosomal recessive trait. Patients homozygous for this allele have a complete absence of arylsulfatase A activity. With the absence of this enzyme, cerebroside sulfate accumulates in the lysosomes of different tissues, including the liver, kidney, gall bladder, and white matter. Deficiency in the activity of this enzyme, the heat-labile component of cerebroside sulfatase, has been established as the primary enzymatic abnormality in MLD.

The deficiency is most frequently demonstrated in urine, peripheral leukocytes, and cultured skin fibroblasts, but is also seen in serum, kidney tissue, and bone marrow cells. Not all of these tissues are affected by the abnormal amounts of this sulfatide, but the white matter of the nervous system does tend to be damaged. In fact, it is the abnormal accumulation of sulfatide within the oligodendroglial and Schwann cells (two cell types found in the myelin sheath) and the metabolic failure of these cells that precede and trigger the events that cause demyelinization. Myelin breakdown results from a defective resorption of cerebroside sulfate, which is necessary for the axon to grow. Additionally, even after maturity, enzymatic failure to metabolize this lipid can prevent normal restructuring of the myelin sheath.

Early on, most patients appear normal clinically and neurologically. Then progressive mental regression, loss of speech, ataxia, and muscle weakness become evident. Genu recurvatum secondary to equinus deformity is often present, and a child who has already learned to walk, similar to the one presented, becomes unsteady in gait.

The child with the late infantile form usually does not survive beyond the first decade. Central and peripheral nervous system demyelinization and degradation often lead to a very debilitating existence, and most of these children contract fatal respiratory infections.

In the present patient, EMG findings were considered to be consistent with a demyelinating neuropathy. MRI findings were consistent with leukodystrophy. These findings, coupled with the discovery of arylsulfatase A deficiency, pointed to the diagnosis. This final stage of metachromatic leukodystrophy proved to be fatal.

Clinical Pearls

1. A complete neurologic examination is imperative when considering any tendon pathology that exhibits either a spasticity or flaccidity.

2. Any change in gait, stance, or position after the child has begun to walk is a cardinal sign of some type of degradation of motor function. A complete exam is required.

REFERENCES

1. Jay RM: Metachromatic leukodystrophy: A case report of a child with an equinus deformity. J Foot Ankle Surg 34:206–207, 1995.
2. Kolodny EH: Metachromatic leukodystrophy and multiple sulfatase deficiency: Sulfatide lipidosis. In Scriver CR, Beaudet AL, Sly WS, Valle D, et al (eds): Metabolic and Molecular Bases of Inherited Disease, 8th ed. New York, McGraw-Hill, 2001.
3. Krivit W: Treatment of late infantile metachromatic leukodystrophy by bone marrow transplantation. New Engl J Med 322(1):28–32, 1990.

PATIENT 24

A 6-year-old boy who walks with flat feet

A 6-year-old boy is seen for evaluation of intoeing. He has been previously diagnosed with bilateral metatarsus adductus. Prior treatment consisted of serial casting for 8 weeks, begun shortly after birth, followed by corrective shoes until age 12 months. His parents feel that the metatarsus adductus has improved since birth; however, they still have concerns about the residual deformity. They deny that their child had any functional problems. Maternal family history is positive for intoeing, which was treated with a Denis Browne bar and corrective shoes.

Physical Examination: Gait analysis: bilateral deformities—rearfoot stance position 20° everted (valgus); forefoot adducted on rearfoot. General (see figure): large prominence at base of 5th metatarsal; prominence of talar head; medial arch thickened with callus over bony prominence. Musculoskeletal: limitation of dorsiflexion at ankle in both knee extension and flexion.

Laboratory Findings: Radiographs: talocalcaneal angle > 35 degrees in the weight-bearing position; lateral subluxation/dislocation of navicular from talar head; adduction of metatarsals at Lisfranc's joint with talar–1st metatarsal angle divergent medially; increased lateral talocalcaneal angle with talus plantarflexed on calcaneus; calcaneal inclination parallel to supporting surface.

Question: What is your concern in a child with recurrent metadductus?

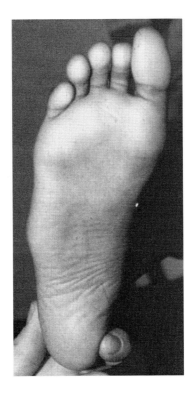

Diagnosis: Residual metatarsus adductus and secondary equinus

Discussion: The position of the navicular on the talar head should be taken into consideration when determining a surgical versus conservative approach. A laterally positioned navicular demonstrates subtalar pronation, while a medially positioned navicular on the talar head is seen with talipes equinovarus and cavus foot deformities. This type of supinated position has to be addressed separately and is usually seen with a forefoot adductus deformity. The radiograph will reveal the navicular position on the talar head. When reducing the metatarsus adductus angle with transverse plane abduction, an abductory force may be exerted at Chopart's articulation. If a lateral deviation of the navicular occurs during this cast reduction, cast therapy should cease. With continued transverse force and midtarsal joint abduction, the result will be a rectus foot at the expense of a pronated flatfoot.

The calcaneal cuboid relationship is studied to determine the presence or absence of forefoot adductus. Forefoot adductus is a soft tissue deformity produced by midtarsal joint supination around the oblique axis, resulting in plantarflexion, adduction, and inversion of the forefoot. Forefoot adductus is evident with an adducted position of the cuboid on the calcaneus. On the radiograph of an adducted forefoot, a line from the calcaneus through the lateral surface of the cuboid deviates in the direction of adduction. Normally, these two lines do not converge. An adducting line demonstrates oblique axis supination; an abducting line demonstrates midtarsal joint oblique axis pronation. In the presence of abduction of the cuboid (midtarsal joint pronation), a metatarsus adductus deformity will need to be addressed more radically and aggressively.

In the present patient, a conservative treatment was planned with the use of a dynamic, stabilizing shoe insert. This orthotic managed his problem successfully by limiting pronatory changes.

Clinical Pearls

1. Total reduction of the metadductus deformity means not just the reduction of the forefoot at LisFranc's, but also prevention of pronation and the development of an equinus. Always reduce the deformity early and maintain in a high flange insert to prevent transverse plane.

2. Equinus is the great deformer of the foot. Consider lengthening procedures, if necessary, to increase dorsiflexion and thus prevent secondary pronation.

REFERENCES
1. Jay RM, Johnson M: Recurrent metatarsus adductus. Current Podiatry 33:33–12, 1984.
2. Kite JH: Congenital metatarsus varus. J Bone Joint Surg 49A:388–397, 1967.

PATIENT 25

A 58-year-old man with complications after arthroplasty

A 58-year-old man was admitted to the hospital with a chief complaint of a stiff, painful first metatarsophalangeal (MTP) joint of the right foot. This condition had been present for many years, but recently the pain become more intense. The patient underwent an arthroplasty of the first MTP joint, with a total silicon–type large implant. He tolerated the surgery, and did not develop any postoperative complications. He was then followed weekly for observation and dressing changes; no complications occurred during this period.

Two months after the surgery, the patient returned with the complaint that the operated MTP joint had become progressively swollen. Warm water soaks were prescribed, along with ampicillin for a 10-day period. Following this therapy, the inflammation decreased. However, a month later, the patient returned to the emergency department with a red, hot, swollen first MTP joint and cellulitis extending proximally to the ankle. The patient was directly admitted to the hospital.

Physical Examinations: *Initial*—Musculoskeletal: MTP joint approximately 10° range of motion; stiff on both plantarflexion and dorsiflexion. Palpation: dorsal prominence; joint painful at rest and upon increased motion. *Late Postoperative*—Skin: slight edema. Palpation: tenderness along MTP joint at surgical site; draining soft-tissue mass on medial aspect of first MTP joint of right foot.

Laboratory Findings: *Initial*—Radiographs (right foot): narrowing and sclerosis of first MTP joint, with mild hallux abducto valgus deformity; small osteophytes and large dorsal ledge on lateral view. *Late Postoperative*—Radiographs (right foot): marked resorption at proximal phalangeal shaft; marked periosteal reaction at first metatarsal shaft and head; radiolucency within shaft and bone at area of total implant.

Questions: What is the most likely diagnosis? What other condition can present with the above findings?

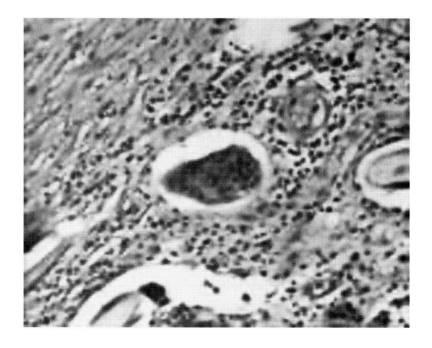

Diagnosis: Osteomyelitis of the first metatarsophalangeal joint with foreign body reaction

Discussion: Silicon is virtually inert; however, there is always the possibility of foreign materials adhering to the implant after autoclaving. The particular matter on the implant—possibly lint from drapes or powder from gloves—is then trapped in the medullary canal and can conceivably touch off a foreign body reaction. When the implant is in place, there is a diminution of the vascular supply to the area in contact with the implant.

With the decrease in blood volume, it is understandable that there will be a decrease in the total phagocytic action in that unit area. Along the same lines, we must consider why there is a predilection of bacteria at the implant site or metaphysis. In the metaphysis, there is a normal slowing down of blood at the juxtametaphyseal hairpin turn. This slowing predisposes a bacterial emboli to settle in the veins and cause thrombosis, with a retrograde occlusion of the capillaries, then transudation, and finally marrow necrosis.

There is also the possibility of avascular necrosis, because capillary loops adjacent to the epiphyseal growth plate are nonanastomising branches of the nutrient artery. Understanding this, we can appreciate the great risk of an insidious contamination or unpredictable infection.

In most noncontaminated surgical wounds, the acute inflammatory reaction subsides, and recognizable tissue repair commences in 3 to 5 days. Surgical wounds that have become contaminated, or those that contain a foreign material not eliminated by the acute inflammatory process, manifest a chronic inflammatory reaction.

Mononuclear cells are the predominant cells of the chronic inflammatory reaction. They phagocytize the remaining foreign material that the enzymes of the granulocytes were unable to make soluble. If the foreign material persists, a chronic inflammatory reaction is set up in which the mononuclear cells undergo a proliferation. These macrophages are responsible for the chronicity of the inflammatory response. They remain in close proximity to the foreign substance for as long as it takes to eliminate it.

The magnitude of a chronic inflammatory reaction depends on both the chemical and physical reactivity of the causative material. Every foreign substance, no matter how inert, evokes an immune response. A relatively inert substance such as silicone, upon removal from the body, might appear as if no reaction had occurred. However, on microscopic examination, a layer of mononuclear cells covered by a thin fibrous capsule is discernible.

In regard to the physical properties of a foreign substance that affect its reactivity, both surface quality and mobility are important. A substance that is smooth and immobile produces much less fibrous proliferation than one that is rough and subjected to motion.

Clinical Pearls

1. Tiny silicone particles can break off an implant with wear or shear within a joint.
2. MRI is most useful to determine the presence of shards within the surrounding joint.
3. Complete removal of the implant should be performed and antibiotics administered prophylactically.

REFERENCE

Shiel WC: Granulamatous inguinal lymphadenopathy after bilateral metatarsalphalangeal joint ailicone Arthroplasty. FootAnkle 6:216–218, 1986.

PATIENT 26

A 19-year-old man with a soccer injury to his right ankle

A 19-year-old man sustained a rapid dorsiflexion injury of the right ankle while playing soccer. He was unable to continue playing because of pain and swelling, which developed rapidly over the next hour. The immediate physical and radiographic examination yielded a diagnosis of a moderate grade II ligamentous sprain of the right ankle. The patient was placed in compressive dressing with a posterior splint, and given crutches with instructions for non-weight bearing. The pain continued for approximately 2 weeks, and the patient felt no better than at the time of original treatment. He now presents for additional assistance.

Physical Examination: Pulses: not palpable due to massive edema. Doppler study: dorsalis pedis and posterior tibial vessels patent. Musculoskeletal: ROM limited and painful in all planes of motion; no pain at medial and lateral malleoli; severe pain upon grasping tibia and fibula malleoli between heels of both hands and squeezing. Pain was greater with subtalar inversion than ankle inversion.

Laboratory Findings: Radiographs: linear, nondisplaced fracture of talar body extending from ankle joint into posterior facet of subtalar joint.

Question: What complication must be ruled out in a patient with a talar fracture?

Answer: Avascular necrosis

Discussion: Talar fractures are relatively uncommon, but they can lead to potentially serious complications. Since the talus has no tendinous attachments, and 70% of its surface is covered by articular cartilage, the blood supply is extremely tenuous. As a result, avascular necrosis (AVN) of the talar body is a common complication.

Although there are a number of classification systems for talar fractures, Canale and Kelly recommend the Hawkins classification. This system describes the fracture pattern and predicts the likelihood of future complications, such as AVN and post-traumatic arthritis. There are four types of fracture with an increasing frequency of AVN: type I has a 0–13% chance of developing AVN; type II is worse, at 20–40%. Type III has a 80–100% chance, and type IV will go on to AVN 100% of the time. The mechanism of injury involves a rapid, forceful dorsiflexion of the foot against a stationary tibia, causing impingement of the talar neck on the tibial plafond. Continued force results in medial and dorsal comminution, along with disruption of the talocalcaneal ligaments and ankle and subtalar capsules. As a result of this disruption, the already tenuous blood supply to the talar body can be significantly disrupted, and AVN occurs.

The diagnosis of AVN can be made on plain radiographic evaluation by the absence of the so-called Hawkins sign. This sign, which Hawkins described as subchondral bony atrophy found in the body of the talus, indicates a normal reactive hyperemic state at 6–8 weeks following these fractures. Additional methods of evaluating AVN include scintigraphy and MRI.

Once AVN has been diagnosed, the goal is to prevent talar dome collapse. According to Penny and Davis, it takes 2 years for a sclerotic talus to revascularize. With this in mind, patients should be kept non-weight bearing on that side for an extended period with the use of a patellar tendon bearing brace.

In the present patient, AVN was ruled out by absence of the Hawkins sign on x-ray. The talar fracture was treated with a below-knee cast, non-weight bearing, for 6–8 weeks.

Clinical Pearls

1. Complications of talar neck fractures include: avascular necrosis (AVN), nonunion, subtalar and ankle joint post-traumatic arthritis, skin necrosis, and osteomyelitis.
2. The first clinical sign of AVN is intractable pain.
3. Evaluate for Hawkins sign 6–8 weeks post-injury.
4. Once AVN is diagnosed, the goal is to prevent talar dome collapse.
5. Revascularization is enhanced by accurate, stable reduction of the fracture fragments.
6. It takes approximately 2 years for a sclerotic talus to revascularize.

REFERENCES
1. Gholan P, et al: Treatment of talar neck fractures: Clinical results of 50 patients. J Foot Ankle Surg 39(6): 365–375, 2000.
2. Penny JN, Davis LA: Fractures and dislocations of the neck of the talus. J Trauma 20:1029–1037, 1980.
3. Thordarson D: Talus fractures. Foot Ankle Clin 4(3):555–570, 1999.

PATIENT 27

A 14-year-old boy with an internal rotation injury to his ankle

A 14-year-old boy is seen in the emergency department after sustaining an internal rotation injury to the right ankle 5 hours ago. Initial treatment consisted of x-rays, ice, elevation, compression bandage, and crutches. The patient was told he had sustained a severe ankle sprain and should remain non-weight bearing for 1 week.

Physical Examination: General: swollen right ankle. Musculoskeletal: pain on palpation of anterolateral aspect of ankle; neurovascular status intact and symmetrical, bilaterally; ankle ROM markedly decreased; pain upon plantarflexion and eversion.

Laboratory Findings: Radiographs: avulsion fracture of tibia on anteroposterior and lateral views. CT scan: intra-articular fracture of epiphysis extending to physis, exiting laterally through open physis, and producing rectangular-shaped fracture. Evaluation revealed a displaced Salter-Harris type III fracture or a juvenile fracture of Tillaux.

Questions: What is the initial treatment of this type of injury? What is the indication for surgery?

Answers: Treatment depends on the amount of displacement. If > 2 mm, surgery is indicated.

Discussion: The mechanism of the juvenile fracture of Tillaux is either a lateral rotation of the foot (abduction) or a medial rotation of the leg on the fixed foot. The fracture fragment is avulsed from the anterolateral aspect of the distal tibial epiphysis by the anteroinferior tibiofibular ligament, when an external rotational force is applied to the foot and reduced by the opposite mechanism. The fracture fragment produced is roughly quadrilateral because the fracture line runs vertically to the physis and exits anterolaterally, producing a Salter-Harris type III fracture of the distal tibial epiphysis.

Treatment is based on the amount of displacement of the articular surface after closed reduction techniques are attempted. If the separation is greater than two millimeters, than arthroscopic-assisted or open reduction with internal fixation is recommended. The prognosis usually is good if anatomic reduction of the articular surface is obtained. The most serious complication reported has been pain and stiffness secondary to articular joint incongruity following inadequate closed reduction.

Initial treatment of a nondisplaced or mildly displaced juvenile fracture of Tillaux should consist of an attempt at closed reduction and placement in a below-knee cast with the foot in internal rotation. In the acute injury, a hematoma block with aspiration of the ankle joint is performed after appropriate skin preparation. The foot is placed in full dorsiflexion and abducted. The mechanism is then reversed with your contralateral thumb applying pressure to the anterolateral tibial physis and fracture fragment. While internally rotating the foot on the leg, maintain axial traction. Anatomical reduction of the fracture fragment is mandatory. If the fracture is displaced more than 2 millimeters, perform open reduction and internal fixation. When the fracture fragment is rotated, closed reduction can be difficult due to interposition of the periosteum and ankle joint capsule.

Surgical reduction requires an anterolateral approach to the ankle joint between and parallel to the extensor digitorum longus tendon and the fibula. Take special care to identify and avoid injury to the lateral cutaneous branch of the superficial peroneal nerve. The superior extensor retinaculum is the first dense structure encountered. When the peroneus tertius is present, the same surgical interval can be used with medial retraction of the tendon. Usually the anterolateral ankle joint capsule is torn along with the syndesmosis, which can lead to instability between the distal tibia and fibula. Inspect the ankle joint to remove any debris. Also check the integrity of the dome of the talus.

With open anatomic reduction of the articular surface, internal fixation is then used to maintain the correction. It is recommended that the internal fixation be placed parallel to the physeal plate, but if it is necessary to cross the physis, smooth Kirschner wires are advised.

In the present patient, open reduction was necessary to reduce the fracture, as displacement was more than 2 millimeters.

Clinical Pearls

1. Attempt closed reduction with compression of the fragment. Take care not to produce a pressure necrosis after the cast has been applied.

2. Inform the patient and family that surgical intervention is usually indicated if the closed reduction has failed (does not appear radiographically).

3. Post-reduction films are indicated to check the reduction. If doubt remains, order CT scans.

REFERENCES
1. Kleiger B, Mankin HJ: Fracture of the lateral portion of the distal tibial epiphysis. J Bone Joint Surg 46A:25,1964.
2. Simon WH, Floros R, Schoenhaus H, Jay RM: Juvenile fracture of Tillaux: A distal tibial epiphyseal fracture. J Am Podiatr Med Assoc 79:295, 1989.
3. Stefanich RJ, Lozman J:The juvenile fracture of Tillaux. Clin Orthop 210:219, 1986.

PATIENT 28

An 11-year-old boy with arch pain

An 11-year-old boy complains of painful arches and increasing discomfort while wearing shoes. His mother observes that his walking has changed, and he cannot run well. He experienced occasional turning in of his ankles over the past year with increasing frequency. The patient's father and paternal uncle had similar problems when they were boys. The child is now seen in the emergency department with a fractured 5th metatarsal base. He states that he was only walking when he felt his foot "give way."

Physical Examination: General (see figure): cavovarus deformities of both feet, with limitation of ankle dorsiflexion; all toes contracted and clawed. Gait analysis: patient unable to walk on heels without balancing himself against wall. Musculoskeletal: muscle strength of tibialis anterior and peroneals weak bilaterally. Neurologic: sensation, particularly vibratory and positional, reduced distally; ankle reflex not elicited.

Laboratory Findings: Electromyographic study: slowed conduction velocities; reduced number of motor unit action potentials and fibrillation potentials; increased proportion of polyphasic potentials and fasciculation potentials.

Questions: What is the diagnosis of this hereditary polyneuropathy? What alternatives are available to allow gait stability?

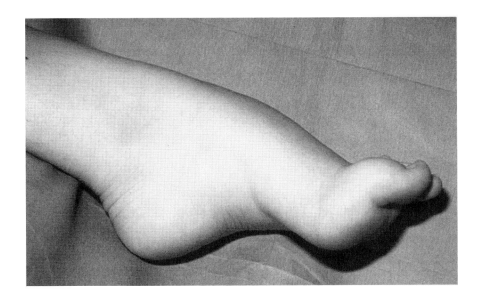

Diagnosis: Charcot-Marie-Tooth disease

Discussion: The prognosis for progression varies with the specific inherited subtype of this polyneuropathy. The inheritance pattern in this case seems to be dominant, implying a better prognosis than if it were recessive.

The first step is to control the rearfoot inversion. Placing the forefoot in valgus minimizes the supinatory rock that will throw the rearfoot into further inversion. The rearfoot can be stabilized with a neutral 0° post to lock the heel; the addition of a high-heeled seat will insure the stability.

In the present patient, a conservative approach was initially taken to manage the progression of the deformity. However, he did not tolerate the orthotics, and surgical options were explored. The surgical procedure consisted of plantar fasciotomy, Dwyer calcaneal osteotomy, tendoachilles lengthening, and posterior tibial transfer through the interosseous space to the dorsum of the foot. The next stage consisted of a Jones procedure to the great toe, proximal first metatarsal osteotomy, and transfers of the extensor tendons into the metatarsal necks. The combination of these procedures reduced the cavus deformity and provided a pain-free gait. The heel varus was reduced, and the ankle spraining was eliminated.

Clinical Pearls

1. A high-flanged, deep heel seat controls the foot and can limit inversion-type injuries.

2. Care must be observed when treating conservatively, as an overposted rearfoot will induce further sprains in the cavus foot.

3. The last resort in children with Charcot-Marie-Tooth disease is a triple arthrodesis; with early recognition, this can be avoided.

REFERENCES

1. Fishman M: Pediatric Neurology. Orlando, Grune and Stratton, 1986.
2. McGlanry E, Banks A, Downey M: Comprehensive Textbook of Foot Surgery, 2nd ed. Baltimore, MD, Williams & Wilkins, 1992.
3. Quin N, Jenner P: Disorders of Movement: Clinical, Pharmacological, and Physiological Aspects. San Diego, Academic Press, 1989.

PATIENT 29

A 72-year-old diabetic woman with a plantar ulcer

A 72-year-old woman is admitted to the hospital with a plantar ulceration of the left foot, located below the 2nd and 3rd metatarsals. Cellulitis on the great toe extends proximally to the 3rd metatarsal. The patient has been diabetic for 15 years, and her diabetes has been controlled with 35 units of insulin NPH. She relates having a bunionectomy 25 years earlier.

Physical Examination: Lower extremity: femoral, popliteal, and dorsalis pedis pulses easily palpable; no redness or swelling; calloused periwound with serous discharge at ulcer site; wound base firm and pink, with granular consistency. Neurologic: no response to Semmes-Weinstein probe.

Laboratory Findings: Chemistries and complete blood counts (including controlled blood sugar): normal. Temperature: 98.6° F. Culture and sensitivity tests of ulcer: no growth on three consecutive samplings. Radiographs (see figure): grossly abnormal left foot—metatarsals tapered absence; 1rst metatarsal neck absent; demineralization and destruction of 2nd metatarsal bone; 1rst metatarsal head and shaft appeared "moth-eaten," with atypical configuration to trabecular structures.

Questions: What is the most likely diagnosis based on the radiographic findings? What methods are used to confirm the diagnosis? Describe the treatment staging that may prevent recurrence of the ulcer.

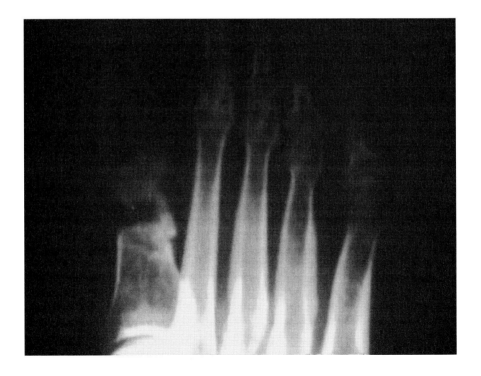

Diagnosis: Osteomyelitis

Discussion: Osteomyelitis associated with peripheral vascular disease, found frequently in diabetics or patients with arteriosclerosis, is a disease of the elderly. The patient with vascular insufficiency of the lower extremity is most likely to develop osteomyelitis from a focus of contiguous infection. Small bones of the feet are most frequently affected, with mixed infection of *Staphylococcus aureus* and enterococci. As would be expected, systemic manifestations are few, and local signs predominate.

Light touch is the primary sense that allows the patient to be aware of and prevent areas of impending breakdown. When this sense is lost, ulceration is inevitable. Therefore, quantifying the pressure sense in a patient's foot is crucial to the exam. The optimal piece of instrumentation to quantify light-touch sensation in a pinpoint distribution adequate for awareness of impending breakdown is the Semmes-Weinstein filament.* This is a nylon probe, smaller than a ball-point pen, that is calibrated to buckle at 10 grams of linear pressure against the patient's skin—the amount of pressure necessary for protective sensation. If the patient cannot feel the probe buckling against the skin, then he or she is at significant risk for the development of neuropathic wounds.

Biopsies and cultures are *not* taken directly from the wound cavity. Wounds are contaminated. Biopsies (bone culture and bone specimen) should be taken from an adjacent, uninfected area via a separate incision.

At the completion of the biopsy, the wound is then addressed by surgical excision. Too often we perform local debridement in the office, removing only the obvious fibrin and necrotic tissue, but leaving devitalized deeper structures. Deep excision of the devitalized tissue to include skin, tendon, muscle, and bone is mandatory. Sharp dissection with a scalpel or with roungeurs of various sizes is helpful in isolating necrotic from healthy tissue. The roungeur is placed underneath the wound edge, and the hyperkeratotic and devitalized tissue is removed.

The 1rst metatarsal head is the most common area for breakdown. The normal foot has an even pattern of motion, with nice, gradual heel contact—a gentle rolling (not excessive) from the outside to the inside of the foot as the foot pronates through, with one bone bearing weight that gradually shifts to another bone.

Contact casting is a way to reduce plantar pressure peaks or the ground reactive pressures, but it does not address shear force. Note that while the cast may be reduce ulceration, upon removal the patient resumes his or her disordered gait pattern, and the shear forces return to create another ulceration in the same or adjacent area.

Osteomyelitis of the 1rst metatarsal head must be addressed with foresight. Understand that the 1rst metatarsal head bears the majority of weight at propulsion, and a resection of the metatarsal will transfer all of the weight to the adjacent metatarsals. The new peak pressure on the 2nd metatarsal head plus the increased shear will lead to future calluses and the potential for plantar ulceration. Carry out a logical sequence when planning metatarsal resections, and consider the deformity in stages:

Stage 1. The infected metatarsal is resected as far proximal as needed, thus decreasing the peak pressure that was the initiating cause of the ulcer. The ulcer is completely and surgically excised, and the patient is placed on appropriate antibiotics determined by bone cultures.

Stage 2. The patient remains 100% off-loaded. Saline dressings, wet-to-dry, are changed twice a day. The dressings should be placed deep into the excised wound cavity.

Stage 3. When the plantar wound has completely closed, the forefoot is addressed with regard to surgical rebalancing. The functional and structural integrity of the forefoot is paramount in reducing the risk of future peak pressure and shear forces related to ulcerations. Rebalancing is performed by panmetatarsal resections, rather than a transmetatarsal or isolated metatarsal resection. The forefoot mechanics are redistributed equally. The weight-bearing surface is spread out transversely over all five metatarsal shafts. With the removal of one metatarsal, increases will occur on adjacent metatarsals.

Stage 4. With the foot now structurally balanced and able to function with equal weight distribution, orthoses can be used. A triple-laminate orthoses not only accommodates the foot by molding and cushioning the abnormal bony prominences, but also supports the foot in a neutral position.

In the present patient, an algorithmic treatment plan was taken to prevent advancement of osteomyelitic progression. The plan involved surgical debridement of the infected bone and soft tissue. The ulcer was surgically excised. The patient was placed on a 6-week course of the appropriate IV antibiotics (determined by the bone cultures).

---

*The Semmes-Weinstein filament can be obtained from the Hansen's Disease Center in Carville, Louisiana. It should be in the armamentarium of all wound-care professionals.

Wet to dry dressing changes were performed twice daily, and she remained non-weight bearing on the affected extremity. Once the wound granulated, the foot was rebalanced with the use of an orthosis to accomodate the abnormal bony prominences and support the foot in a neutral position. The patient has now returned to normal daily activities.

Clinical Pearls

1. Never perform swab cultures of a wound; they are all contaminated, but not all are infected.
2. Bone biopsies and bone cultures are the gold standard in the diagnosis, and mandatory in setting up the proper course of antibiotic and surgical treatment.

REFERENCES

1. Bell JA: Light-touch, deep-pressure testing using Semmes-Weinstein monofilaments. In Mackin EJ, Callahen AD, Osterman AL, et al (eds): Rehabilitation of the Hand, 5th ed. St. Louis, Mosby, 2001.
2. Waldvogel FA, Medoff G, Swartz MN: Osteomyelitis Clinical Features, Therapeutic Considerations, and Unusual Aspects. Springfield, IL, Charles C Thomas, 1971.
3. Weingarten MS: The Management of the Chronic Non-Healing Wound. Philadelphia, Graduate Hospital Wound Care Center educational manual, 1992.

PATIENT 30

A 65-year-old, insulin-dependent woman with a painful blister

A 65-year-old insulin-dependent woman presents with a painful "blister" on her right foot. She states that it appeared very rapidly, and has not responded to oral antibiotics and local wound care. It is quite painful upon pressure. The woman is wearing sneakers and socks. There is no history of lengthy walks or running that may have caused the blister.

Physical Examination: Temperature 99.6° F; vital signs stable. General: alert and well oriented to surroundings. Lower extremity: dorsalis pedis and posterior tibial pulses steady and palpable. Skin (see figure): no trophic changes other than a 2.5-cm erythematous ring with a 1-cm central bullous eruption, located centrally on dorsum of right foot. Musculoskeletal: area surrounding raised mass quite tender upon palpation.

Laboratory Findings: WBC 16,200/μl; ESR 160 mm/hr; fasting glucose 180 mg/dl. Culture from bullae: negative for aerobe, anaerobe, fungal, and AFB.

Question: What is your clinical impression?

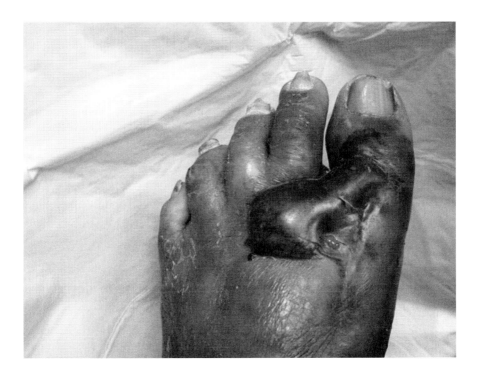

Diagnosis: Pyoderma gangrenosum

Discussion: Pyoderma gangrenosum (PG) was first described by Brusting, Goekerman, and O'Leary in 1930 as a rare, destructive, reactive neutrophilic dermatosis. PG begins as tender papules or vesicles, which develop into painful ulcerations surrounded by induration and erythema.

Pyoderma gangrenosum ulcers may exhibit pathergy, which is an exaggerated response to a minor trauma and can lead to expansion of the ulceration. PG can be iatrogenically induced from vaccination, injections, and surgery. Therefore, surgical debridement is a direct contraindication in this condition.

PG most commonly affects the lower extremities; however, there is an atypical form of the disease that is more prevalent in the upper extremities, head, and neck. PG primarily affects young to middle-aged adults and is seen more frequently in women then men.

Diagnosis of PG, according to Bennett et al., is a diagnosis of exclusion, and there is no specific laboratory or histopathologic test. Biopsy of the ulceration will likely show epidermal ulceration with adjacent epidermal hyperplasia. Dermal inflammatory infiltrates and vessel walls with fibrinoid necrosis are also seen histologically.

PG can be associated with several systemic diseases. The literature states that inflammatory bowel disease and arthritis are the most commonly reported disease associations, followed by hematologic malignancy. PG has also been associated with diabetes, SLE, HIV, and many other conditions.

The treatment of PG has been extensively debated. Topical therapy for mild conditions can include corticosteroid agents to the borders of the lesion, hydrocolloid dressings, antibacterial agents, and compression and elevation of the affected limb. Nonimmunosuppressive agents such as Dapsone and clofazimine have also been used in the treatment of PG. The most commonly used and successful therapy is oral corticosteroids in large doses. Prednisone (1–2 mg/kg) is used for moderate to severe PG. However, high doses of prednisone can be accompanied by hypertension, hyperglycemia, osteoporosis, and increased susceptibility to infection.

The present patient's blister eventually ruptured and developed into an ulceration with surrounding erythema. Cultures revealed no growth. A biopsy of the lesion revealed dermal inflammatory infiltrates with fibrinoid necrosis of vessel walls and epidermal ulceration with adjacent hyperplasia. A course of local wound care and topical corticosteroids to the borders of the lesion was initiated. The lesion began to respond quickly to therapy. An Apligraft allogenic skin graft was applied to the base of the wound to increase healing time and decrease wound contracture. The patient had immediate relief of painful symptoms. After a 1 month course of therapy, the wound was 100% epithelialized. She has had no recurrence of ulcerations.

Clinical Pearls

1. Initial presentation of a painful, sterile nodule that eventually ulcerates is a key in the diagnosis of pyoderma gangrenosum.
2. When performing the aspirate, it is wise to collect a tissue sample at the same time. Try to include the inner surface of the bullae or the base.
3. The hemorrhagic appearance is the salient feature of the disease.
4. Appearance is a severe destructive state.

REFERENCES

1. Bennett ML, Jackson JM, Jorizzo JL, et al: Pyoderma gangrenosum: A comparison of typical and atypical forms with an emphasis on time to remission. Case review of 86 patients from two institutions. Medicine 79(1):37–46, 2000.
2. Burr BS: The etiology and treatment of leg ulcers. J SC Med Assoc 89:67–70, 1993.
3. Imus G, Golomb C, Wilkel C, et al: Accelerated healing of pyoderma gangrenosum treated with bioengineered skin and concomitant immunosuppression. J Am Acad Dermatol 44:61–6, 2001.

PATIENT 31

A 23-year-old woman with excruciating foot pain after a motorcycle accident

A 23-year-old woman arrives at the emergency department via ambulance complaining of excruciating right foot pain. She has just been in a motorcycle accident. She was hit head-on by another vehicle and sustained a severe dorsiflexion injury to her right ankle. She also has a minor laceration to the face, but denies any other pain.

Physical Examination: Vital signs: stable. HEENT: normal. Cardiac: regular rate and rhythm; mild tachycardia. Chest: clear. Abdomen: benign. Skin: normal; no attenuation or breakdown. Neurologic: motor and sensory intact. Lower extremity: right ankle and foot in guarded position of slight plantarflexion; dorsalis pedis and posterior tibial pulses strong. Musculoskeletal: gross swelling of midfoot and ankle, with ecchymosis; marked tenderness about ankle joint and subtalar joint, with decreased ROM and crepitus.

Laboratory Findings: CBC: normal. Radiographs: skull, spine, and chest—no abnormalities. Ankle lateral view (see figure)—talus posteriorly displaced, with vertical fracture through neck; dislocation of subtalar joint; ankle and talonavicular joint intact. Urinalysis: normal.

Questions: How is this fracture classified? What is the most common complication?

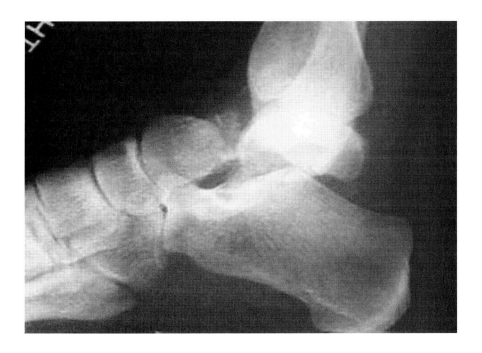

Diagnosis: Talar neck fracture, Hawkins type II

Discussion: The talus bone is primarily cancellous, with no muscular origins or insertions, and two-thirds of the surface area is covered with articular cartilage. Therefore, a high percentage of talus fractures are intra-articular, and, due to the tenuous blood supply, avascular necrosis is a common complication.

Three main branches supply blood to the talus: the posterior tibial, anterior tibial, and peroneal arteries. The posterior tibial artery is further divided into the calcaneal, supplying the posterior tubercle; artery of the tarsal canal, supplying the body; and deltoid, supplying the medial side of the talus. The anterior tibial artery branches into the medial tarsal, supplying the superior medial neck; lateral tarsal, supplying the talar head; and artery of the sinus tarsi, which supplies the talar neck and body and is formed by anastomosis between the lateral tarsal and perforating peroneal.

The typical talar neck fracture is vertical from the dorsal neck and exits the tarsal canal, which is the weakest portion of the talus. There are two theories as to the mechanism of injury: a hyperdorsiflexion causes the neck to impact against the anterior edge of the distal tibia, or the talus acts as a cantilever and the neck breaks due to bending forces. The most widely used classification system for talar neck fractures is the one developed by Hawkins in 1970:

Group I—undisplaced vertical neck fractures

Group II—displaced fractures with subtalar joint dislocation

Group III—displaced fractures with subtalar joint and ankle dislocation

Group IV—displaced fractures with subtalar joint, ankle, and talonavicular dislocation.

Most talar neck fractures, except nondisplaced, require open reduction with anatomic alignment and insertion of a lag screw.

Avascular necrosis (AVN) is likely to occur if two-thirds of the blood supply is disrupted, causing weakening of the talar trochlea, which is subject to collapse if full weight-bearing is allowed. The incidence of AVN is around 40% for a type II injury and 90–100% for type III and IV fractures. Radiographic presentation may occur at 1–4 months, appearing as a relative increase in bone density due to loss of blood supply and no bone resorption. The surrounding bone becomes osteoporotic as a result of reactive hyperemia from trauma; disuse is also a factor. The presence of subchondral atrophy (lucency) in the dome of the talus on an AP radiograph (**Hawkins' sign**) is indicative of healing and viability. The atrophy, which usually occurs at 6–8 weeks, results from disuse osteopenia and vascular congestion, suggesting continuity of blood supply.

Treatment of AVN includes nonweight-bearing cast immobilization with anatomic union for up to 2 years or arthrodesis, such as subtalar, triple, pantalar, or tibiocalcaneal (Blair fusion).

In the present patient, an extremely conservative approach was taken. She was cast for 12 weeks, and then used a Cam walker for 3 months. She was kept nonweight-bearing the entire time. No radiographic changes were noted, and the patient continued with the Cam walker for an additional 3 months. Her talus did not collapse, and a treatment of external fixation of the ankle along with pulsed electromagnetic field stimulation was attempted. Evidence of revascularization was noted, and the patient underwent a pantalar fusion using an iliac graft to maintain loss of the extremity length. These procedures were successful in returning her to full mobility.

Clinical Pearls

1. Neck fractures are the second most common talar fracture and occur from either a hyperdorsiflexion or the talus acting as a cantilever.

2. The blood supply to the talus, which is very rich but extremely delicate, comes from three main sources: posterior tibial, anterior tibial, and peroneal arteries.

3. Hawkins' classfication of talar neck fractures comprises four groups, based on increasing dislocation of surrounding joints.

4. Avascular necrosis is the most common complication. It appears radiographically as a relative increase in bone density.

5. Hawkins sign is indicative of viability. It presents at 6–8 weeks and appears radiographically as a subchondral lucency.

REFERENCES

1. Canale TS, Kelly FB: Fracture of the neck of the talus: Long-term evaluation of 71 cases. J Bone Joint Surg 60A:143–156, 1978.
2. Metzger MJ: Talar neck fractures and rates of avascular necrosis. J Foot Ankle Surg 38(2):154–162, 1999.

PATIENT 32

A 34-year-old woman with high-arched feet and ankle pain

A 34-year-old woman presents with bilateral ankle pain. She relates aching pain in her lateral ankles that worsens with increased activity, and complains of frequent ankle sprains. She states that she has always had very high-arched feet and has difficulty wearing certain shoe gear. The patient denies any trauma. She has tried prefabricated orthotics with little relief.

Physical Examination: Vital signs: stable. HEENT: normal. Cardiac: regular rate and rhythm. Chest: clear. Abdomen: benign. Skin: normal. Neurologic: diminished deep tendon reflex, decreased vibratory sensation. Musculoskeletal: flexible, bilateral cavovarus deformity with plantarflexion of 1st ray; evidence of weakness with resistive ROM of tibialis anterior; contracture of lesser digits with hyperkeratotic lesions at dorsal PIP joint; no instability of ankles; no tenderness along lateral ligaments; atrophy of posterior leg muscles.

Laboratory Findings: CBC with differential: normal. Nerve conduction velocities: 50% decrease in motor and sensory velocity, 25 m/sec, distal latencies delayed. Radiographs (see figure): marked calcaneal inclination, with divergence of talar neck in plantarflexion; talocalcaneal angle 0° on AP view.

Questions: What is the diagnosis? What are some treatment options?

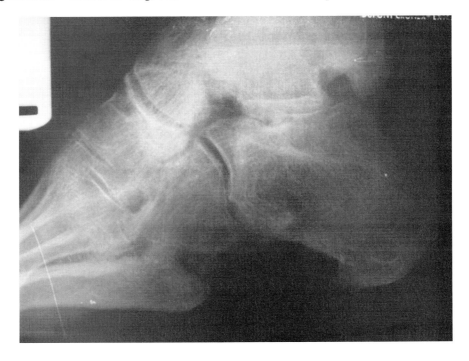

Diagnosis: Charcot-Marie-Tooth (CMT) disease

Discussion: CMT disease is a hereditary motor and sensory peripheral neuropathy resulting from an abnormality of myelination. It accounts for 90% of all hereditary neuropathies. Charcot and Marie of France and Tooth of England described it simultaneously in 1886. Originally the disease was described as a peroneal muscle atrophy, but it was determined later that the peroneals maintain most of their strength until the late stages of the disease.

There are two types of CMT. Type I or hypertrophic CMT is the classic presentation. It is usually autosomal dominant and begins in the third decade of life. Type I progresses slowly, with demyelination and atrophy of nerve fiber causing moderate impairment of muscle function. Type II or nonhypertrophic is the neuronal form, with symptoms less pronounced and occurring later in life. The pathophysiology of the hypertrophic form involves abnormal enzymes and molecules along the nerve causing premature atrophy. There is a remyelination and onion bulb effect that causes enlargement of the nerve. The nonhypertrophic form shows neuronal atrophy with no evidence of demyelination.

Clinical manifestations include distal muscle atrophy and weakness—usually bilateral and symmetrical—of the upper and lower extremities. Muscle degeneration follows a specific pattern. The muscles supplied by the longest axons of the sciatic nerve are affected first, and the smallest muscles are the first to atrophy. Common presentation also includes cavovarus and equinovarus foot type, contracture of lesser digits, drop foot, and/or a steppage gait. The cavovarus deformity is due to weakness of the tibialis anterior and peroneus brevis, causing the peroneus longus to plantarflex the 1rst ray, resulting in a forefoot valgus. The remaining metatarsals may also be plantarflexed, causing soft tissue contracture at the metatarsophalangeal joint and dorsal subluxation of the digits. The unopposed pull of the posterior tibialis exaggerates the hindfoot varus. There is also some level of sensory loss; vibratory sense and proprioception are affected first.

The Coleman block test is used to determine the flexibility of the rearfoot with a plantarflexed 1rst ray. A wooden block is placed underneath the lateral border, and heel and rearfoot pronation is evaluated. If the rearfoot corrects to neutral or valgus, then a 1rst ray procedure will reduce the hindfoot deformity. If the rearfoot fails to move, a midfoot or hindfoot procedure is warranted.

Diagnostic studies include nerve conduction velocities, EMG, DNA analysis, and nerve biopsy. Nerve conduction velocities are often 50% reduced in motor and sensory conduction, and distal latencies are two to three times more than normal.

Conservative treatment consists of extra-depth shoes, accommodative orthotics, and strengthening and stretching exercises. Surgical treatment can be very complex; three questions should be answered before a procedure is done.

1. What is the motor status of the muscles around the foot and ankle?
2. Is the deformity flexible or fixed?
3. How extensive is loss of sensation?

The selection of surgical procedure depends on your answers to these questions, the patient's age, and the chief complaint. Surgical correction includes arthroplasty or arthrodesis of lesser digits; dorsiflexory osteotomies of metatarsals; peroneus longus or posterior tibial tendon transfer; midfoot osteotomies (Cole or Japas); calcaneal slide osteotomy; or, for a severe varus, a Dwyer osteotomy. Triple arthrodesis should be used as a salvage procedure for a long-standing, fixed deformity with signs of hindfoot degenerative changes. The key to a successful procedure is relocating the calcaneus beneath the talus, causing valgus of the hindfoot and allowing the talus to plantarflex.

In the present patient, conservative therapy was attempted. Custom-molded orthoses were constructed with deep heel cups to maintain control of the rearfoot. The forefoot was rebalanced to accommodate the forefoot valgus. The patient had a significant decrease in lateral ankle pain and denied any further ankle sprains at a 6-month follow-up appointment. Continuous monitoring for evaluation of the progression of the disease is done monthly. At this time, she is still functioning without difficulty.

Clinical Pearls

1. Charcot-Marie-Tooth disease is a hereditary, progressive motor and sensory neuropathy that comprises a hypertrophic type and a nonhypertrophic type.

2. CMT usually presents with a cavovarus deformity, sensory loss, contracture of digits, and atrophy of lower extremity muscles ("stork leg" appearance).

3. Both motor and sensory conduction velocities are 50% reduced.

4. Use the Coleman block test to determine the flexibility of the rearfoot.

5. Surgical principles include correcting fixed deformities, restoring muscle balance, and preventing recurrence.

6. Radiographic features include dorsiflexion and abduction of the talus on the calcaneus ("bullet-hole sinus tarsi"), increased calcaneal inclination, and plantarflexion of the 1st ray.

REFERENCES

1. Fishman M: Pediatric Neurology. Orlando, Grune and Stratton, 1986.
2. Quin N, Jenner P: Disorders of Movement: Clinical, Pharmacological and Physiological Aspects. San Diego, Academic Press, 1989.

PATIENT 33

An 11-year-old girl with a short toe

An 11-year-old girl presents with concern about abnormal toes and, more specifically, pain in her right fourth toe. The mother states that her daughter has been complaining of discomfort, which is aggravated by wearing sneakers, for approximately 2 weeks. Most of her pain is located in the center of the forefoot. In addition, the child's activity level is notably decreased. Around the age of 4 or 5, the girl's 4th toes were noted to be short and deformed. There is no history of injury or trauma. Past medical history is unremarkable, with no known drug allergies. Family history is positive for hypertension and diabetes mellitus.

Physical Examination: Vital signs: normal. Pulses: palpable dorsalis pedis and posterior tibial bilaterally. Neurologic (lower extremity): normal. Dermatologic: no skin lesions; skin texture and turgor normal. Musculoskeletal: bilateral 4th toe dorsal dislocation, with shortening of 4th toe; mild bilateral hallux abducto valgus deformity with flexible pes planus; limited plantar flexion ROM of 4th metatarsophalangeal joints bilaterally.

Laboratory Findings: Radiograph (see figure): short 4th metatarsal of both feet; no joint changes at 4th metatarsophalangeal joint.

Question: What is this anomaly commonly referred to as?

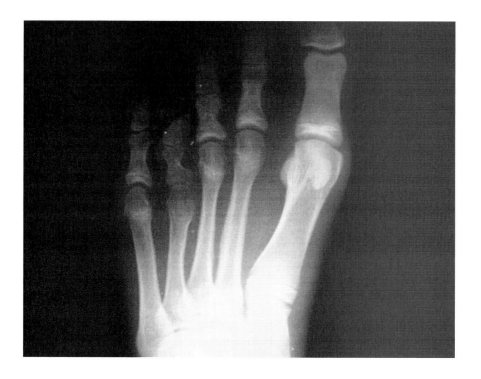

Diagnosis: Brachymetatarsia

Discussion: Brachymetatarsia is character-ized by an abnormally short metatarsal bone. The condition is primarily hereditary in nature and although it predominantly affects the fourth metatarsal bone, it may affect multiple metatarsals. The shortening of the metatarsal is due to prema-ture closure of the epiphyseal line at the distal por-tion of the metatarsal. Although the etiology is unknown, brachymetatarsia has been associated with Down's syndrome, pseudohypoparathy-roidism, pseudo-pseudohypoparathyroidism, Al-bright's syndrome, Turner's syndrome, dias-trophic dwarfism, and other systemic disorders. Brachymetatarsia is more common in females (2.5:1) and most often occurs bilaterally. Radi-ographic evaluation is used to confirm an osseous shortening of the metatarsal.

In the early stages of development, patients are usually asymptomatic. The primary complaint in the younger patient is often cosmetic, and many times these patients are self-conscious about their appearance. Older patients may experience symp-toms of pain due to excessive pressure under ad-jacent metatarsal heads; clinically one may see callus formation in these areas. Skin, soft tissue, and tendon contractions lead to additional dis-comfort with use of shoes.

Treatment of brachymetatarsia may include conservative care, such as an orthotic device to re-distribute pressure away from adjacent metatarsal heads. Shoe gear may be modified to accommo-date the dorsally located digit. Definitive treat-ment requires surgical correction to address the soft tissue contractions as well as the shortened metatarsal. Numerous surgical procedures exist to correct brachymetatarsia, including bone grafts, metatarsal osteotomies, distraction osteogenesis with external fixation devices, and tendon length-ening and skin plasty techniques to address the soft tissue contractions.

In the present patient, callus distraction (cal-lotasis) was performed by gradually lengthening the metatatarsal, creating osteogenesis between the two bone fragments.

Clinical Pearls

1. Brachymetatarsia is an anomaly, often congenital, that causes a shortened metatarsal and floating toe.

2. Brachymetatarsia predominantly occurs in females, with a 2.5:1 female to male ratio.

3. Cosmetic and psychological complaints may present early, followed by painful calluses and difficulty wearing shoes as the deformity progresses.

4. Conservative treatment may be more appropriate in certain patients, but surgical correction is the definitive treatment.

REFERENCES
1. Choi IH: Metatarsal lengthening in congenital brochymetatarsia: One-stage lengthening versus lengthening by callotasis. J Pediatric Orthop 19(5):660–4, 1999.
2. Kite JH: The Clubfoot. Grune and Stratton, New York, 1964.

PATIENT 34

A 25-year-old man with persistent ankle pain

A 25-year-old man presents with a chief complaint of persistent left ankle pain of 9-month duration. He states that the pain developed while he was participating in a recreational football game. He denies any history of direct trauma to the area. Treatment with ice, aspirin, and compressive ACE bandages has offered minimal relief of symptoms.

Physical Examination: Vital signs: normal. Vascular: 2/4 dorsalis pedis and posterior tibial arteries bilaterally; immediate capillary refill. Neurologic: epicritic sensation in lower extremity intact bilaterally; negative Tinel's sign on percussion of tibial nerve. Skin: texture and turgor normal; no edema or erythema. Musculoskeletal: normal ankle, subtalar, and midtarsal ROM; no evidence of pain on passive joint mobility; positive pain with active plantarflexion and eversion; mild pain on palpation of left Achilles tendon; moderate to severe pain on palpation between Achilles and peroneal tendons, posterolateral to the subtalar joint.

Laboratory Findings: Radiographs: accessory bone posterolateral to talus on lateral view of left foot.

Question: What is the likely diagnosis of this patient's persistent ankle pain?

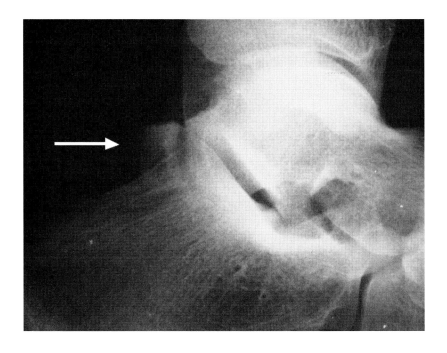

Diagnosis: Os trigonum syndrome

Discussion: Numerous accessory bones may be located throughout the foot. The os trigonum is an accessory bone posterolateral to the talus. The talus has two posterior tubercles, medial and lateral. In some cases, the lateral process may be elongated, in which case it is termed Steida's process. With severe ankle plantarflexion, the lateral tubercle may also fracture when impacted between the tibia and calcaneus, and thereby imitate an os trigonum. Differentiation of an os trigonum and a fractured lateral talar process can be difficult. A fracture is usually more irregular in shape and has sharp edges; an os trigonum generally has smoother borders. Typically the os trigonum ossifies between ages 8 and 11 and may be seen on a lateral ankle radiograph.

Clinically, a painful os trigonum may present as diffuse posterior ankle pain, which increases with activity. The flexor hallucis longus tendon courses between the posterior talar tubercles, and when the hallux is dorsiflexed, the patient's pain may be reproduced. Ligamentous attachments may also place stress on the area, creating pain with ankle dorsiflexion. Biomechanically, both supinated and hyperpronated feet can cause os trigonum syndrome. MRIs and CT scans are aids to diagnosis.

Treatment may be conservative, consisting of nonsteroidal anti-inflammatory drugs, local corticosteroid injection, ankle supports/braces, orthotic devices, and/or immobilization with a below-knee cast. If conservative treatment fails to alleviate symptoms, surgical excision of the os trigonum may be necessary.

In the present patient, the os trigonum was surgically excised via a medial approach.

Clinical Pearls

1. Os trigonum syndrome is a condition of pain experienced upon irritation of an accessory bone posterolateral to the talus.

2. Clinically an os trigonum may lead to similar symptoms as that of a fractured posterolateral talar tubercle.

3. Conservative treatment should be employed initially. If symptoms persist, surgical excision of the bone should relieve symptoms.

REFERENCES
1. McGlamry ED, et al. Comprehensive Textbook of Foot Surgery, 2nd ed. Baltimore, Williams & Wilkins, 1992.
2. Moeller FA. The os trigonum syndrome. J Am Podiatr Assoc 63:491–501, 1973.

PATIENT 35

A 46-year-old woman with a lump on the top of her foot

A 46-year-old, otherwise healthy woman presents with the chief complaint of a painful, soft tissue lump on the top of her right foot. She states that the mass appeared approximately 3 weeks ago and has progressively become larger. Wearing shoes causes increased pain and discomfort, with occasional numbness felt around her lateral digits. The patient denies a history of trauma.

Physical Examination: Vital signs: normal. Pulses: 2/4 dorsalis pedis and posterior tibial bilaterally, with immediate capillary refill. Neurologic (lower extremity): epicritic sensation intact bilaterally; positive Tinel's sign with percussion of intermediate dorsal cutaneous nerve. Skin: texture and turgor normal; no erythema or edema; 2-cm diameter, raised, soft tissue mass on dorsal lateral aspect of right midfoot, underlying extensor brevis muscle; mass freely movable and transluminates light. Musculoskeletal: ankle, subtalar, midtarsal, and metatarsophalangeal joints ROM normal; mild pes planus deformity bilaterally.; muscle strength 5/5 bilaterally.

Laboratory Findings: MRI (see figure): signal changes under extensor digitorum brevis and travels into subtalar joint. Radiographs: no osseous changes.

Question: What is your diagnosis?

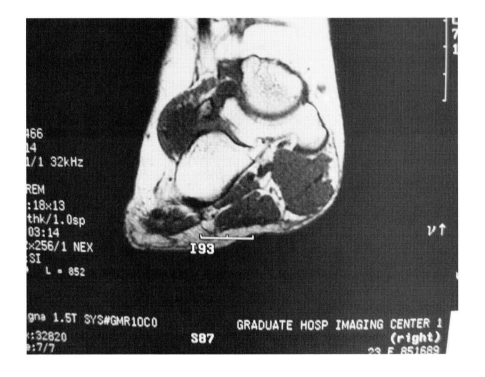

Diagnosis: Ganglion

Discussion: Ganglia are relatively common soft tissue lesions. They are defined as cysts containing mucopolysaccharide—rich fluid within fibrous tissue or, occasionally, muscle, bone, or a semilunar cartilage. The cyst usually occurs adjacent to a joint or in tendon sheaths and most often in repetitively traumatized areas. Ganglia have also been referred to as myxoid cysts, peritendinitis serosa, or synovial cysts. The dorsal aspect of the foot is a common location for development of a ganglion, and tight shoe gear may play an important role.

Treatment of ganglia includes needle aspiration, infiltration of corticosteroid, padding and mild compression, and surgical excision. Ganglia can recur, and may require surgical excision if symptoms persist.

In the present patient, needle biopsy confirmed the diagnosis. The ganglion was situated directly under the extensor digitorum brevis (see figure, *top*), with the stalk leading into the subtalar joint (see figure, *bottom*). The lesion continued to recur despite numerous aspirations. When excised, the ganglion was located around the medial dorsal cutaneous nerve, which was dissected free and protected. The hypertrophic bone at the 1st metatarsal-cuneiform joint was resected to further reduce irritation of the area postoperatively. The patient was asymptomatic at 6 months, with a negative Tinel's sign.

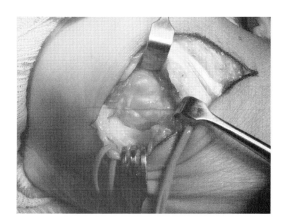
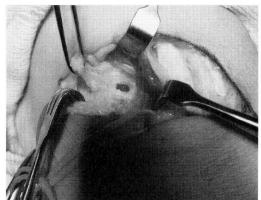

Clinical Pearls

1. A ganglion often forms on an area of irritation, overlying a joint or connected to a tendon sheath.

2. A common location is the dorsum of the foot, but ganglions may occur anywhere on the foot.

3. Needle aspiration, padding, and compression may relieve symptoms, but if the ganglion persists and creates pain and discomfort, perform surgical excision.

4. Ganglions are well-defined masses that transluminate within the soft tissue.

5. Aspiration of a ganglion reveals a straw- or amber-colored liquid.

REFERENCES

1. Banks AS, Downey MS, Martin DE, Miller SJ : McGlamry's Comprehensive Textbook of Foot and Ankle Surgery, 3rd ed. Philadelphia, Lippincott, Williams & Wilkins, 2001.
2. Stedmans Medical Dictionary, 27th ed. Philadelphia, Lippincott, Williams & Wilkins, 2000.

PATIENT 36

A 26-year-old man with a painful, discolored great toenail

A 26-year-old man presents with a complaint of pain in his right great toe. Yesterday he played in a long tennis match, during which he had considerable discomfort. He also relates that he was wearing a new pair of tennis sneakers. Following the match, he noticed discoloration of his great toenail along with a localized, throbbing pain. The pain became progressively worse over the next 12 hours despite ice and ibuprofen. It was localized to the medial aspect of the great toe, and was aggravated with shoe gear and simple ambulation. The patient's past medical history is unremarkable, and he denies previous injuries to his feet.

Physical Examination: General: no acute distress; well developed, well nourished. Cardiac: normal. Chest: clear bilaterally. Neurologic: normal. Lower extremity: right hallux nail discolored medially; mild erythema along proximal/medial nail margin. Skin: no open lesions. Vascular: status intact. Orthopedic: no gross deformity. Musculoskeletal: considerable pain with palpation, especially along proximal medial border of nail.

Laboratory Findings: Radiographs: no evidence of distal tuft fracture or associated fractures.

Question: What is your diagnosis based on this clinical presentation?

Diagnosis: Subungual hematoma

Discussion: Subungual hematomas result from repetitive digital microtrauma. Compression of the nailbed between the nailplate and the underlying distal phalanx can damage nailbed arteries. There is a potential dead space between the nail plate and the underlying nail bed and matrix, which then fills with blood. Subungual pressure secondary to this hemorrhage can damage matrix cells and the surrounding healthy nail bed, and often causes extreme pain.

Patients typically present with a swollen toe and complaints of throbbing pain following a digital injury. The two most common mechanisms are repetitive microtrauma from sports such as tennis, and a crush-type injury. The hemorrhagic nail plate discoloration usually confirms the diagnosis. It is important, however, to obtain radiographs of the digit since approximately 20–25% of subungual hematomas are associated with an underlying phalangeal fracture.

Treatment involves drainage of the blood to reduce subungual pressure. Hematomas involving less than 25% of the nail plate are usually drained with trephination. Commonly used techniques include a heated paperclip, an 18-gauge needle, and a hand-held electrocautery device. Once the plate is penetrated, the blood collection is expressed with slight pressure. The area should then be cleansed and dressed with a dry sterile dressing.

When the hematoma involves more than 25% of the nail plate, there is an increased risk of nail bed laceration. In fact, 60% of hematomas covering more than 50% of the nail plate are associated with nailbed lacerations that require repair. As a result, complete avulsion to evaluate the entire nailbed is recommended in these instances.

Decompression of a subungual hematoma is quick, easy, and painless. Patients feel immediate relief and generally have no complications following prompt drainage. Automatic nail avulsion typically occurs within 6 weeks, and a new nail has usually regrown by 6 months without dystrophy.

In the present patient, a no. 11 scalpel blade was used in a drilling fashion to drain the hematoma from beneath the nail. The patient immediately had relief of the pain.

Clinical Pearls

1. Fractures are associated with 20–25% of subungual hematomas.
2. Nail bed lacerations must be considered when the hematoma involves > 25% of the nail plate.
3. Subungual hematomas are caused by microtrauma and by crush injuries.
4. Hand-held cautery is ideal for trephination.
5. Prompt decompression is important.
6. Hutchinson's sign must be ruled out.

REFERENCES

1. Malay S. Trauma to the nail and associated structures. In McGlanry ED, Banks A, Downey M (eds): Comprehensive Textbook of Foot and Ankle Surgery, 2nd ed. Baltimore, Williams and Wilkins, 1992.
2. Pearson A, Wolford R. Management of skin trauma. Prim Care 27(2), 2000.

PATIENT 37

A 36-year-old woman with left forefoot pain after a jog

A 36-year-old woman presents with complaints of pain in the area of her left forefoot. She first had discomfort in this area 4 weeks ago following a jog with a friend. The pain was initially more of a generalized ache that would come and go with her workouts, but it gradually became more intense with activity, despite rest. Persistent discomfort began affecting simple ambulation. The patient was seen in a local emergency department 2 weeks ago, where x-rays were read as negative. Since then she has tried ice and heat, as well as aspirin for pain, without relief.

The patient has jogged two to three times a week for the past 2 years. She also relates a recent increase in her mileage. Her past medical history is significant for hypertension and gastric ulcerations. She has no other complaints at this time and, besides the aspirin, is taking only Toprol XL.

Physical Examination: General: normal appearance, no recent weight change. Cardiac: normal. Chest: CTA bilaterally. Neurologic: no focal defects, CN 2–12 intact. Lower extremity: flexible pescavus foot type with mild gastrocnemius soleus equinus bilaterally. Vascular: normal. Skin: left forefoot edema and ecchymosis; no open lesions. Musculoskeletal: no pain with dorsiflexion and plantarflexion at the 2nd MTP joint; no pain with MTP joint compression/distraction; negative Mulder's sign; pain on palpation of distal aspect of 2nd metatarsal shaft and at 3rd metatarsal head with plantar to dorsal pressure. No pain with vibratory stimulation of third metatarsal. No obvious clinical deformity noted.

Laboratory Findings: Radiograph (see figure): exuberant bone callous proximal to anatomical neck at 2nd metatarsal; intracortical lucency medially; alignment acceptable.

Question: What is your diagnosis?

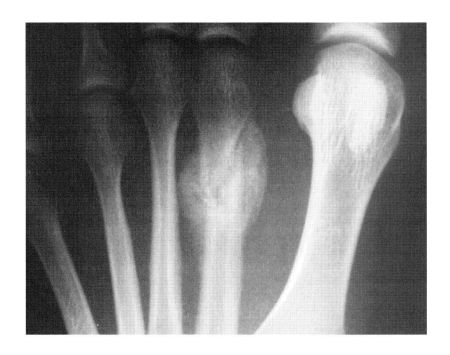

Diagnosis: Second metatarsal stress fracture

Discussion: Briethaupt was the first to describe metatarsal stress fractures, in 1855. They were commonly seen in young military recruits, which led to the term "march fractures." Today, these fractures usually result from overuse and are seen most commonly in the female athletic population.

Women are less able to absorb shock due to a wider pelvis (coxa vara/genu valgum) and 25% less muscle mass. They also have a lower bone mineral density, especially post-menopause. The "female athlete triad" for stress fractures includes: eating disorders, amennorhea, and osteopenia.

Structurally, while a cavus foot is more likely to lead to a tibial stress fracture, planus feet are more prone to metatarsal stress fractures. Additionally, those with metatarsus primus elevatus, Morton's foot, or leg length discrepancy are also at increased risk. Hyperpronation as well as conditions such as hallux limitus/rigidus can increase the stress on the 1st and 2nd metatarsals. While equinus has not been found to be a significant risk factor, most feel that a rear foot inversion greater than 33 degrees increases the risk of developing metatarsal stress fractures. Extrinsic risk factors include training errors, footwear, the surface or terrain, and individual fitness levels.

Ninety percent of metatarsal stress fractures affect metatarsals 2–4, typically occurring in the distal third of the shaft. An exception to this rule is found in ballet dancers who sustain proximal fractures near the tarsometatarsal joint (secondary to "en pointe" postures). There is also a high incidence of 2nd metatarsal stress fractures after 1st ray surgery (especially Keller's procedure).

Radiographically, 30–70% of metatarsal stress fractures initially appear normal. Positive findings typically become apparent by 3 weeks, but may take up to 6 weeks. A linear cortical lucent region associated with periosteal and endosteal thickening is seen in diaphyseal bone. A focal sclerosis (band-like condensation of trabeculae) is seen in metaphyseal bone. The gold standard for diagnosis is a triple-phase bone scan. Although nonspecific, this test is very sensitive and is usually positive within 24–48 hours of the injury.

The differential diagnosis includes: metatarsalgia, neuroma, neuritis, pre-dislocation syndrome, capsulitis, and bone tumor. A complete clinical history and thorough physical exam will usually lead to an appropriate diagnosis. Most patients relate an insidious onset of pain, with gradual progression of symptoms. Often, there is an associated recent increase in activity level. On physical exam the hallmark is pinpoint tenderness. Forefoot edema, pain with passive dorsiflexion, as well as an inability to hop on the affected foot are classic findings.

Once a diagnosis has been made, treatment usually begins with RICE principles. Conservative care with immobilization (surgical shoe), and partial weight bearing is often effective. A gradual return to activity is very important, and swimming is often an excellent start. Remember, as with any fracture, complete healing will take 4–8 weeks.

In the present patient a wedge shoe was dispensed to off-load the forefoot. This approach combined with the other conservative principles mentioned above led to uneventful healing.

Clinical Pearls

1. Ninety-five percent of stress fractures occur in the lower extremity.

2. The risk of stress fracture in women is 2–10 times the risk in men.

3. Patients relate an insidious onset of pain with gradual progression. On physical examination, the hallmark is pinpoint tenderness.

4. Initial radiographs frequently do not reveal the fracture; 30–70% are normal. Repeat radiographs during weeks 2–3 will reveal a bone callus at the site of the stress fracture.

5. The diagnostic gold standard is a triple-phase bone scan.

6. A gradual return to activity is a must!

REFERENCES
1. Kaufman KR, et al. The effect of foot structure and range of motion on musculoskeletal overuse injuries. Am J Sports Med 1999; 27(5).
2. Mandelbaum BR, et al. Stress fractures. Clin Sports Med 1997; 16(2).

PATIENT 38

A 61-year-old man with soft tissue masses at his ankle and heel

A 61-year-old man presents with relatively painless soft tissue masses on the posterior aspect of his left heel and ankle. He has a long-standing history of seropositive rheumatoid arthritis (RA). Although these nodules initially appeared over 2 years ago, they have grown considerably during the past 3 months. The patient was diagnosed with RA 15 years previous. He was effectively treated with NSAIDs for most of that time, until an acute rheumatoid flare prompted the addition of methotrexate. He has been maintained on a low dose of methotrexate (7.5 mg/week), along with various NSAIDs (currently Celebrex). The patient also relates recent worsening of his generalized morning stiffness.

Physical Examination: General: well developed, well nourished; ambulatory. HEENT: negative for scleritis, oral lesions, and thyromegaly; neck supple. Cardiac: normal. Chest: clear bilaterally. Neurologic: no focal defects, CN 2–12 intact. Skin: no rashes. Upper extremity: MCP swelling, mild boutonnière deformities digits 2 and 5 bilaterally. Lower extremity: soft tissue nodules on posterior aspect of left heel and ankle measuring 3.5 × 2 × 1 cm and 2 × 1 × .5 cm, respectively; no lesser digital contractures; mild bilateral hallux abducto valgus deformity. Vascular: normal.

Laboratory Findings: ESR 32 mm/hr, rheumatoid factor 704. Radiographs: soft tissue densities; no evidence of calcaneal erosion; mild joint space narrowing without erosions.

Question: What is your diagnosis, based on this clinical presentation?

Diagnosis: Rheumatoid nodules

Discussion: Rheumatoid arthritis is a chronic, polyarticular, symmetric, inflammatory disease with a predilection for small proximal joints. Currently affecting 2.5 million Americans, this disease strikes women three times more often than men. Although the characteristic feature of RA is inflammatory synovitis, multiple extra-articular organ systems can be affected. In general, the number of these complications increases with disease severity.

The most frequently recognized skin lesion in RA is the rheumatoid nodule. These nodules usually develop during an active phase of the disease and have been reported to occur in 20–30% of patients with RA. Patients who develop rheumatoid nodules commonly have severe RA, and almost invariably are seropositive (+RF).

Rheumatoid nodules are usually located in superficial subcutaneous tissue, but can occur in deeper structures such as bursa, joints, tendons, or ligament. They are found on periarticular structures, extensor surfaces, and other areas subjected to mechanical pressure. Common locations include the olecranon bursa, the sacrum, the occiput, and the Achilles tendon. They usually present clinically as firm, flesh-colored, nontender, and freely moveable masses. Histologically, rheumatoid nodules are granulomatous lesions characterized by areas of central necrosis. The periphery is composed of palisading fibroblasts and histiocytes with chronic inflammatory infiltration.

The pathophysiology behind rheumatoid nodules is not completely understood, but a few theories have been postulated: (1) vascular inflammatory changes followed by necrosis, (2) repetitive microtrauma, and (3) genetic factors, specifically the HLA-DR B1 04 alleles. Additionally, it is well accepted that methotrexate, which has become the gold standard of RA therapy, can cause an accelerated nodulosis.

The differential diagnosis includes ganglions, gouty tophi, abscess, and xanthomatosis. If after a careful history and clinical examination there is still a question as to the diagnosis, an excisional biopsy can be performed. This however, is rarely necessary. Although these nodules are most commonly seen with RA, they can also be seen in other chronic inflammatory disorders such as systemic lupus, granuloma annulare, and necrobiosis lipoidica diabeticorum. In these cases the history becomes extremely important in making a correct diagnosis.

Rheumatoid nodules are usually nontender and often regress completely with time. However, they can become sources of continued irritation. Complications, such as overlying skin breakdown with secondary infection and/or underlying bony erosion, can also occur. Conservative measures of treatment include aperture padding, intralesional steroid injections, and colchicine. With the ability to inhibit giant cell formation, colchicine has been found to gradually reduce rheumatoid nodules. If these conservative measures fail, surgical excision becomes necessary.

In the present patient, the nodules became quite large and created pain with all shoe gear. It was decided to surgically excise them.

Clinical Pearls

1. Only 1% of all rheumatoid nodules occur in the feet. Common locations are the olecranon bursa, sacrum, and Achilles tendon.
2. Rheumatoid nodules usually indicate an advanced disease state.
3. Histologic features include a central necrosis rimmed by palisading fibroblasts.
4. Local trauma can be a precipitating event. Methotrexate may accelerate nodulosis.
5. Nodules often regress or involute spontaneously.
6. Colchicine may help reverse these growths.

REFERENCES

1. Anderson R: Rheumatoid arthritis. Primer on the Rheumatic Diseases, 11th ed. Atlanta, GA, Arthritis Foundation, 1997.
2. Patton J, et al: Rheumatoid arthritic foot. J Am Podiatr Med Assoc 83(5):270–275, 1993.
3. Sanders, Timothy. Rheumatoid Nodule of the Foot: MRI appearances mimicking an indeterminate soft tissue mass. Skel Radiol 27: 457–460, 1998.
4. Williams F, et al: Accelerated cutaneous nodulosis during Methotrexate therapy in a patient with rheumatoid arthritis. J Am Acad Dermatol 39(2): 359–362, 1998.

PATIENT 39

A 29-year-old man with a painful ankle

A 29-year-old man presents to the emergency department (ED) after being struck by a motor vehicle. He is experiencing pain and swelling of the right foot and ankle, and is unable to bear weight on the right. He denies any other complaint or area of tenderness. The patient relates that while he was crossing the street and stepping onto the curb, a passing car traveling at approximately 20 mph struck the outside of his right leg/ankle. He attempted to walk, but was unable to put any pressure on his right foot/ankle. He was immediately taken to the ED for evaluation.

Physical Examination: Temperature: afebrile. Vital signs: stable. HEENT: normal. Chest: clear. Cardiac: regular. Abdomen: nontender. Skin: superficial abrasion on lateral aspect of right leg, with mild ecchymosis of medial heel and ankle. Neurovascular status: intact. Musculoskeletal: pain on palpation to lateral leg and medial ankle, with mild associated edema; painful active and passive ROM of right ankle; zero pain on palpation to right foot; also no pain at ankle level on lateral compression of fibula.

Laboratory Findings: Radiographs: *Right foot*—no osseous pathology; no fracture or dislocation. *Right ankle* (see figure)—transverse proximal/midshaft fibula fracture without displacement, angulation, or shortening; distal oblique medial malleolar fracture of tibia, with medial and plantar migration of distal fragment; increase in medial clear space.

Questions: What is the mechanism of injury? How would you treat the fracture?

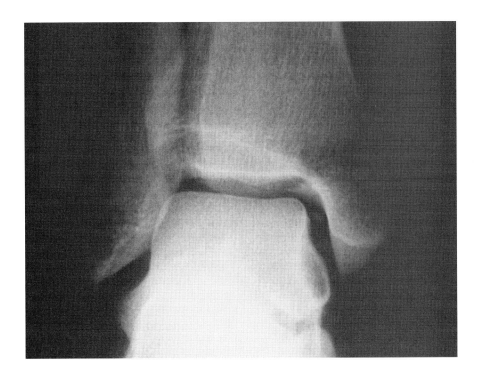

Diagnosis: The mechanism was trauma (a direct blow) without any rotational forces.

Discussion: Ankle injuries are one of the most common injuries seen in the ED. Whether the injury is diagnosed as an ankle sprain, strain, fracture, or fracture/dislocation, a thorough understanding of the mechanism of injury will allow the clinician to properly treat the disorder. Some difference of opinion exists as to whether ankle injuries should be x-rayed in the ED. If there is a possibility of a fracture or if the patient is unable to bear weight on the extremity, than a radiograph should be obtained.

When evaluating an ankle fracture, the physician must evaluate both soft tissue and osseous derangement. Having a working knowledge of the pathological forces that caused the fracture will facilitate accurate anatomical joint restoration. In the present patient, displacement of the medial malleolar fracture and an increase in the medial clear space led to the decision to perform an open reduction with rigid internal fixation (ORIF). The ORIF was performed to regain stability of the ankle joint and to anatomically reduce the fracture, while at the same time providing the patient with the best long-term outcome.

The ORIF was done to his medial malleolar fracture only. The decision to conservatively manage his high fibula fracture was based on the already near-perfect alignment of the fibular fracture fragments and the *non*disruption of the interosseous membrane and anterior inferior tibiofibular ligament. This injury resulted from a direct trauma/ blow to the right leg and ankle. The high fibular fracture did not result from a pronation or eversion injury; therefore, a transsyndesmotic screw or repair of the anterior inferior tibiofibular ligament was not indicated or necessary.

The medial malleolar fracture was fixated with two 4 × 40 mm, parallel, partially threaded, and cannulated screws through a curvilinear incision over the distal aspect of the tibia under C-arm direction (see figure). Once the medial malleolar fracture was properly reduced, the ankle mortise and fibular fracture were again evaluated under fluoroscopy. The medial clear space was reduced; no tibiofibular diastasis was noted on ankle ROM; and the fibular fracture remained in excellent alignment. The patient was then immobilized in a below-the-knee cast. Weight bearing and physical therapy were initiated after the cast was removed, at approximately 6 weeks.

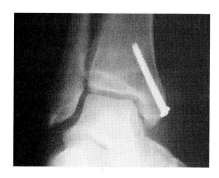

Clinical Pearls

1. A high fibular fracture is usually associated with an eversion or pronation type of movement of the foot upon the leg.

2. Proximal fibula fractures typically have an associated anterior inferior tibiofibular ligament and interosseous membrane rupture, which are usually primarily repaired and fixated with a transsyndesmotic, fully threaded cortical screw.

3. Medial malleolar fractures can be repaired percutaneously under fluoroscopy guidance or opened and reduced with two parallel cancellous or partially threaded cannulated screws to anatomically align the fracture and to prevent rotation.

4. The focus on surgical correction of ankle fractures is to restore the length of the fibula, assure syndesmotic stability, and accurately realign the ankle mortise.

5. Osteochondral defects of the talus often occur with fracture-dislocation injuries about the ankle.

REFERENCES

1. Banks AS, Downey MS, Martin DE, Miller SJ : McGlamry's Comprehensive Textbook of Foot and Ankle Surgery, 3rd ed. Philadelphia, Lippincott, Williams & Wilkins, 2001.
2. Mitchell M, Howard B, Sartoris D, Resnick D: Radiologic review: Diagnostic imaging of trauma to the ankle and foot: 1. Fractures about the ankle. J Foot Surg 28: 174–179, 1989.
3. Reinherz R, Granoff S, Henning K, Ross B: Characteristics of operative management of supination external rotation: Ankle fractures. J Foot Ankle Surg 30(4): 356–363, 1991.

PATIENT 40

A 21-year-old woman with a stiff, painful foot

A 21-year-old, otherwise healthy woman presents with a 4-month history of acute left rearfoot pain. The patient also relates a chronic discomfort in her left foot since early childhood; this discomfort was remitting in nature and nonprogressive until recently. She describes her symptoms as a dull ache with occasional periods of sharp, shooting pain, which limit her weight-bearing activities. She denies any history of trauma, but has been more active due to nursing school rotations and waitressing duties the past several months. Previous treatment consisted of plantar heel injections, stretching and strengthening exercises, custom-molded orthotics, and NSAID therapy without any major relief in symptoms. Her condition is particularly aggravated after strenuous activity, and is relieved only with long periods of rest.

Physical Examination: HEENT: normal. Chest: clear. Cardiac: regular. Abdomen: nontender. Skin: normal texture/turgor/temperature; no ecchymosis; mild pitting edema of left lateral rearfoot and ankle. Musculoskeletal: pain on palpation to left lateral midfoot, rearfoot, and ankle; ROM of left ankle normal; ROM of left subtalar joint (STJ) significantly decreased and extremely painful on both inversion and eversion; ROM of left midtarsal joint mildly decreased, but without discomfort; left forefoot normal.

Laboratory Findings: Radiographs: moderate degenerative changes in STJ, with joint space narrowing and surrounding increased sclerosis; jagged appearance of sustentaculum tali; midtarsal joint congruent and without arthritic degeneration. MRI (see figure): increased signal intensity on T2-weighted image in area of sinus tarsi, most likely related to bone marrow edema defusing out from adjacent talus and calcaneus; irregularity at articulating aspect of STJ, particularly at middle facet, representing predominately cartilaginous communication with some interposed osseous formation on T1-weighted image.

Question: What is the most likely cause of the patient's decreased ROM and pain in the rearfoot?

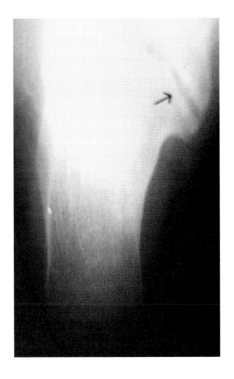

Diagnosis: Subtalar joint coalition (middle facet)

Discussion: Generalized pain, discomfort, and stiffness in the hindfoot and ankle area has many causes, and the differential diagnosis can be extensive. A thorough history and physical exam, as well as the use of radiographic modalities such as plain-film radiography, MRI, CT scan, and even a three-phase bone scan, can help narrow your differential.

Tarsal coalition is a foot condition in which a bridge or bar across two or more tarsal bones limits or eliminates motion between the involved bones or joint. The etiology of is still unclear, but the disorder may be acquired or congenital. A coalition can be a syndesmosis (a fibrous union), a synchondrosis (a cartilaginous union), a synostosis (an osseous union), or any combination of the three.

Tarsal coalition is sometimes accidentally found on routine radiographs, and the patient may be completely asymptomatic. However, if symptoms are present they usually consist of diffuse pain, muscle spasm, and limitation of joint motion. The pain onset is typically insidious, or it can occur abruptly as a result of minor trauma. Symptoms are usually aggravated by activity and relieved with rest. The symptoms of a middle facet talocalcaneal coalition present as pain localized to the sinus tarsi laterally and the sustentaculum tali medially, and as a significantly decreased STJ range of motion.

Conservative treatment usually consists of NSAIDs, physical therapy, injections, below-knee casting, and orthotics, particularly those that restrict subtalar and midtarsal motion. Orthotics are most effective when manufactured to hold the rearfoot in a neutral or valgus position. If conservative therapy fails, then surgical intervention is necessary to relieve symptoms. Surgical treatment essentially involves fusion of the involved joint complex or resection of the bar with or without performing an adjunctive procedure.

Clinical Pearls

1. A middle subtalar joint (STJ) coalition is considered to be the most common tarsal coalition found in the foot.

1. MRI and CT scan are extremely useful imaging modalities if there is a high suspicion of a tarsal coalition, especially when x-rays are inconclusive.

2. The symptoms of an STJ or midtarsal joint coalition are aching and stiffness, particularly in the region of the sinus tarsi or deep in the STJ.

3. Peroneal spastic flat foot can be a sequela of a tarsal coalition, in which the rearfoot becomes fixed in a rigid valgus position.

4. The results of bar resection are poor when degenerative adaptations have occurred in the area of coalition or surrounding joints of the rearfoot. A primary fusion of the STJ or midtarsal joint may be necessary to relieve symptoms.

REFERENCES

1. Alter S, McCarthy BE, Mendicino S, DiStazio J: Calcaneonavicular bar resection: A retrospective study. J Foot Ankle Surg 30(4): 383–389, 1991.
2. Stoller MI: Tarsal coalition—A study of surgical results. J Am Podiatr Assoc 64: 1004–1015, 1974.
3. Swiontkowski MF, Scranton PE, Hansen S: Tarsal coalitions: Long-term results of surgical treatment. J Pediatr Orthop 3: 287–292, 1983.

PATIENT 41

An 84-year-old man with painful hallux ulcers

An elderly gentleman presents with extremely painful ulcers on his hallux and toes. They have developed over 6 months, and are not responding to conservative treatment. The patient has a history of noninsulin-dependent diabetes, peripheral vascular disease, coronary artery disease, congestive heart failure, and atrial fibrillation.

Physical Examination: General: well appearing; no apparent distress. Temperature 98.2°, blood pressure 140/65, pulse 64, respirations 12. Skin (see figure): ulcers of right second toe and hallux; erythema of entire forefoot; ulcers dry with a pale-colored granulation tissue; 100% fibrin covering on these wounds, which measure 18 mm × 12 mm × 3 mm; tip of right hallux gangrenous, no drainage. HEENT: pupils 3 mm equal and reactive; moist mucous membranes without lesions; dentition poor; neck without bruits or lymphadenopathy. Chest: clear. Cardiac: no jugular venous distention; regular rate and rhythm; systolic ejection murmur. Abdomen: positive bowel sounds, without distention or tenderness; no organomegaly. Rectum: negative, without polyps or prostate abnormality. Extremities: bilateral femoral and popliteal pulses without distal pulses.

Laboratory Findings: Dipyridamole MIBI test: anteroseptal defect with partial perfusion consistent with myocardial infarct. Noninvasive vascular testing: no left dorsalis pedis Doppler wave form. Left ankle/arm index 0.56. Radiographs (of digits): no any evidence of osteolysis or osteomyelitis. Arteriogram: stenosis at distal femoral artery and blockage just proximal to trifurcation; good flow to dorsalis pedis, but no flow to digits.

Question: What is your clinical diagnosis?

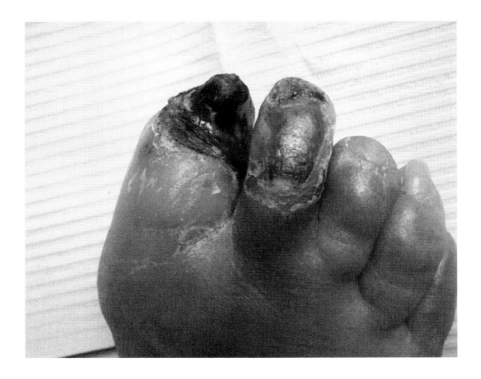

Diagnosis: Arterial occlusive disease

Discussion: Obviously, a bypass of the blockage should be considered. The question is what to do with the foot in light of the patient's age and medical status. The patient was determined to be an Anesthesia Class III according to ASA physical status classification reported by Sakladin in 1941. Cardiac catheterization prior to any planned surgery was recommended. A femoral distal popliteal reversed saphenous vein bypass graft, under spinal anesthesia, is recommended. This procedure will increase pressures to the foot, but will not revascularize the digits. A plan for a Lisfranc's proximal amputation should be considered at the same time as the bypass. This will capture the best time for a patent vessel and minimize the risks of anesthesia. The patency of the distal arteries within the foot will dictate whether the Lisfranc amputation site should be distal or proximal.

Clinical Pearls

1. Decide at the time of revascularization whether to close or leave the amputation site open.

2. All too often, the distal flow is not strong enough, and necrosis of the flap closing the site leads to an abscess. When in doubt, leave the amputation site open.

3. Leaving a wound open for delayed closure is a viable option for the surgeon. Wet to dry saline packing is advisable. Once the bed has granulated sufficiently, the wound can be closed; if complete closure does not occur, consider growth factors to accelerate healing.

REFERENCES

1. Campbell DR: Diabetic vascular disease. In Frykberg: The High-Risk Foot in Diabetes Mellitus. New York, Churchill Livingstone, 1991, pp 33–38.
2. Pinzur M: Amputation level selection in the diabetic foot. Clin Orthop 296:68–70, 1993.

PATIENT 42

A 55-year-old woman with a raised mass on her second toe

A 55-year-old woman presents with a swollen lesion around her right second toe. It has been increasing in size over the past 6 months. Over the previous 4 weeks, the mass became painful with ambulation. The patient cannot recall any history of trauma or stepping on an object. Her past medical history is unremarkable, except for slight obesity. She denies taking any medications, and is in good physical health.

Physical Examination: General: raised mass on plantar aspect of second metatarsophalangeal joint, measuring 25 mm diameter and 13 mm height; firm and fluctuant; not painful upon compression between examiner's thumb and forefinger; no redness.

Laboratory Findings: Radiographs: soft-tissue swelling with no osseous involvement. Histopathology: bulbous, lobular, gray soft-tissue mass excised from plantar aspect of right foot was demonstrated to be a cyst with numerous giant cells and abundant keratin.

Question: How did this lesion develop?

Diagnosis: Epidermal inclusion cyst with foreign-body giant-cell reaction

Discussion: Epidermal inclusion cysts usually occur secondary to traumatic implantation of epidermal cells into dermal tissue. Once in the deeper subcutaneous tissues, the epidermal cells grow, producing a lipid- and keratin-filled cyst that can enlarge and become quite painful and sometimes infected. Epidermal inclusion cysts create a foreign-body giant-cell reaction; this inflammation may lead to the formation of a sinus tract. When squeezed, a sinus tract yields a cheesy exudate consisting mainly of keratin.

Treatment of this lesion is excision of the cyst and sinus tract. Left untreated, a rare occurrence of malignant transformation of epidermal cells may occur.

In the present patient, an epidermal inclusion cyst developed despite the absence of a history of stepping on a sharp object. Oftentimes these lesions develop from repetitive trauma, such as with ill-fitting shoe gear, as was the case in this patient. Radiographs are helpful in determining osseous extent. In the present patient, because there was no osseous involvement, the cyst was excised, and she made a full recovery.

Clinical Pearls

1. Epidermal inclusion cysts usually occur secondary to trauma; without this history, rule out ill-fitting shoes as etiology.
2. Excise the lesion, as it is possible for these masses to become malignant.

REFERENCES

1. Delacretaz J: Keratotic basal-cell carcinoma arising from an epidermoid cyst. J Derm Surg Oncol 3: 310–11, 1977.
2. Potter GK, Ward KA: Tumors. In McGlamry ED, Banks AS, Downey MS (eds): Comprehensive Textbook of Foot Surgery, 2nd ed. Baltimore, Williams and Wilkins, 1992, pp 1139–1140.

PATIENT 43

A 2-year-old girl with one severely flattened foot

A 2-year-old girl is brought in by her mother for an evaluation of her right foot. The mother is concerned because "it looks different than the other foot." The child was delivered full term in a small hospital by the local family doctor. This is her very first physical exam. She is the mother's third child; the two other children have no lower extremity pathology and are quite healthy. The remainder of the girl's history is normal, except for the lack of recent and required vaccinations.

Physical Examination: General: right foot appears shorter than left, and is positioned up and outward in reference to leg (see figure). Large prominence on inner aspect of foot. Convex deformity of plantar aspect of foot with heel in valgus. Musculoskeletal: limitation of dorsiflexion at ankle, leaving foot in equinus; talar head felt on medial plantar aspect of foot; forefoot abducted and dorsiflexed at midtarsal joint.

Laboratory Findings: Radiographs (standing AP and lateral, lateral plantarflexion, lateral dorsiflexion): increased talocalcaneal angle with forefoot abduction; calcaneus in equinus with vertical position of talus; dorsal displacement of forefoot on talus; line bisecting talus did not pass through longitudinal axis of metatarsals—was malaligned in both lateral and lateral plantarflexion views (see figure).

Questions: What is your diagnosis? What are some treatment options?

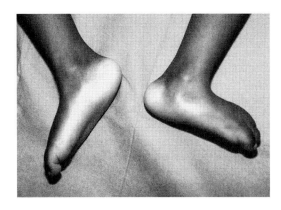
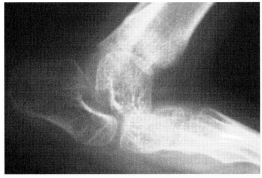

Diagnosis: Vertical talus

Discussion: The synonyms for vertical talus are: congenital convex pes valgus, congenital flatfoot with talonavicular dislocation, and congenital rigid rocker-bottom foot. The etiology is unknown. There is a high incidence in various congenital anomalies and neuromuscular diseases, such as myelomeningocele, congential dysplasia of the hip, arthrogryposis, trisomy 13–15, and Marfan's syndrome. Both males and females are equally affected, but right foot involvement is slightly higher.

The condition is classified according to mobility and presence of the above findings:

Group I: supple feet that resemble calcaneovalgus feet; radiograph needed to make the diagnosis

Group II: rigid feet; sometimes part of a syndrome

Group III: vertical talus associated with trisomy 13–15 or 18

Group IV: vertical talus associated with neuromuscular problems such as spina bifida.

Anatomically, the calcaneus is in valgus and equinus, with no anterior talocalcaneal articulation. The talus is fixed in a vertical position, with associated hypoplasia of the talar head and neck. The navicular articulates with the dorsal cortex of the talar neck. The tibionavicular and dorsal talonavicular ligaments are contracted, precluding reduction of the navicular on the talus. A contracted calcaneocuboid ligament causes forefoot abduction, and the posterior capsule and subtalar joint are contracted. Muscle and tendons of the anterior tibial, extensor hallicus longus, extensor digitorum longus peroneal, and Achilles are all contracted. The posterior tibial tendon as well as the peroneal tendons are anteriorly displaced.

The treatment goal is to reduce and maintain the anatomic relationship of the navicular and calcaneus to the talus. Casting should be started at birth and continued for 3 to 4 months, to stretch the soft tissues in preparation for future surgery. Reducing the talonavicular dislocation will eliminate forefoot valgus. The foot is positioned for cast application by holding the forefoot in equinus and varus. The rearfoot is supinated and held in dorsiflexion and inversion.

Conservative treatment is usually unsuccessful, especially if it is started late. Surgical procedures include soft tissue release with posterior capsulotomy, tendon lengthenings (extensor hallucis longus, extensor digitorum longus, peroneal, and Achilles tendons), and tendon transfers (split ATT and peroneal tendon). These soft-tissue procedures may provide an incomplete reduction of deformity, and bony procedures, including excision of navicular, talecomy, and subtalar/triple arthrodesis, have to be considered.

In the present patient, the plan was to restore the bone and joint relationship. A two-stage approach was taken: First, the extensor digitorum brevis was resected from its origin, and the sinus tarsi was evacuated. Lengthenings were performed on the tibialis anterior, extensor hallucis longus, and extensor digitorum longus. The talonavicular joint was mobilized and maintained with K-wire fixation. This position was held for 6 weeks in an above-the-knee cast. The second stage consisted of removing the pins and lengthening the tendoachilles. The tibialis anterior was translocated, and the foot and leg were immobilized. After cast removal, the child was maintained in a DSIS insert.

Clinical Pearls

1. Early recognition (at birth) of vertical talus is critical.

2. Casting should be performed for a minimum of 3 months. Even if it doesn't completely reduce the deformity, it will minimize the surgical procedures needed.

3. Pinning the first ray, reducing the abduction, and realigning the talus can provide good early reduction of the deformity.

REFERENCES

1. Benard MA: Congenital vertical talus. Clin Podiatr Med Surg 17(3):471–80, 2000.
2. Drennan JC, Sharrard WJW: The pathological anatomy of convex pes valgus. J Bone Joint Surg (Br) 53:455–461,1971.
3. Kumar SJ, Ramsy PL: Vertical and oblique talus: A diagnostic dilemma. Orthopaedic Transcriptions 1:108,1977.
4. Tachdijian MO: Congenital convex pes valgus. Orthoped Clin North Am 3:131–148,1972.

PATIENT 44

A 10-year-old boy with a painful right arch

A 10-year-old boy presents with a painful right arch. He started noticing the pain about 3 days earlier and feels most of it along the top of his foot, especially when he is walking or running. There is minimal discomfort at rest. His mother does not know of an injury to the foot, but she has noticed that he feels warmer at night and may be running a fever. The child has not been out of the city in 2 years and plays locally.

Physical Examination: General: essentially normal health, with no other joint or bone pain. Temperature: 39.1° C. Musculoskeletal: acute pain over base of first metatarsal; mild swelling in this area.

Laboratory Findings: WBC 14,500/µl, increased polymorphonuclear leukocytes, ESR 50 mm/hr (normal 0–20). Aspiration in region of first metatarsal base: positive for *Staphylococcus aureus*. Radiographs: no abnormalities of foot; epiphyseal plates open with no signs of fractures or dislocation. Bone scan: increased uptake in right first metatarsal, with predominant uptake in epiphyseal region, as compared to left, unaffected side; focal increase in epiphysis of right first metatarsal proximally on delayed images (again compared to left).

Question: What is your diagnosis?

Diagnosis: Subacute epiphyseal osteomyelitis

Discussion: Factors that influence infective processes in bone include host resistance, virulence of the bacteria, trauma creating a vascular injury, and ischemia in the bone. *Staphylococcus aureus* is the most common organism seen in hematogenous osteomyelitis, and *S. aureus* has been found to have a certain affinity for the epiphyseal margins. The blood supply to the epiphyseal end is through a tortuous and juxtapositional artery that gives off branches to the metaphysis and epiphysis. These arteries form very narrow and more tortuous turning arteries, making hairpin turns that eventually slow the blood. This is similar to the effect of a highway reducing the number of lanes in a turn: the traffic slows or even stops. Thus, bacteria can lodge within the loops at the epiphyseal junction.

The blood supply in the venous loops is analogous to the sluggish flow in the metaphysis, which is the site of acute hematogenous osteomyelitis. The two conditions are quite similar in presentation, and treatment is dependent upon the radiographic findings. If lucency is seen in the bone ends near the epiphysis, curettage of the bone is indicated. With the absence of bone changes, IV antibiotic therapy alone is sufficient.

In the present patient, IV coverage was sufficient to eradicate the infection.

Clinical Pearls

1. In light of the pain and lack of trauma in subacute epiphyseal osteomyelitis, it is important to set up a differential diagnosis with the use of x-ray, CT scan, and MRI.

2. Include the following in your differential diagnosis: osteogenic sarcoma, chondroblastoma, Ewing's sarcoma, unicameral bone cyst, Brodie's abscess, and osteoid osteoma.

3. Whether curettage and antibiotics or a sole course of treatment with antibiotics is instituted, stabilization of the foot is paramount.

REFERENCES

1. Letts RM: Subacute osteomyelitis of the growth plate. In Behavior of the Growth Plate. London, UK, Raven Press, 1988.
2. Lindenbaum S, Alexander H: Infections stimulating bone tumors: A review of subacute osteomyelitis. Clin Orthop 184:193, 1984.
3. Ross ERS, Cole WG: Treatment of subacute osteomyelitis in childhood. J Bone Joint Surg 67-B:443, 1985.

PATIENT 45

A 30-year-old man with a clinically deformed left foot and ankle

A 30-year-old man presents to the emergency department with a painful, edematous, clinically deformed left foot and ankle. He fell off his bicycle during a professional BMX (bicycle) race, and now relates a mechanism of plantarflexion/inversion. He complains of severe pain and mild paresthesias in the foot, and is unable to bear any weight on that side. The patient has no complaints of head, neck, or back pain and denies any loss of consciousness or nausea. Past medical history is unremarkable, and he is taking only ibuprofen on an as-needed basis.

Physical Examination: Temperature 99° F, BP 134/86 mm/Hg, heart rate 68 bpm, respirations 15. General: alert and oriented to person, place, and time; well developed, well nourished. HEENT: head contusions; pupils equal, round, and reactive to light and accomodation; extraocular muscles intact; visual acuity intact. Pedal pulses: 1/4 dorsalis pedis, 2/4 posterior tibial. Vascular: capillary fill time 3–5 seconds. Skin: no open lesions, no fracture blisters; lateral aspect of foot and ankle extremely edematous and ecchymotic; tenting of skin of mid foot level. Neurologic: epicritic sensation intact; mild paresthesias distally. Musculoskeletal: guarding and weakness upon plantarflexion and dorsiflexion; inability to invert or evert; foot in position of severe inversion, plantarflexion, and adduction, with dorsal lateral prominence at mid foot level; mild tenderness to palpation over medial malleolus; severe pain along dorsal mid foot and 5th metatarsal.

Laboratory Findings: Radiographs: < 25% talonavicular apposition, with medial displacement of calcaneus; multiple associated fractures—lateral navicular, medial talar dome, post talar process, and 5th metatarsal.

Question: What is your diagnosis?

Diagnosis: Medial subtalar joint dislocation with associated fractures

Discussion: DuFaurest and Judcy first reported subtalar dislocations in 1811. By definition this injury involves a simultaneous dislocation of the subtalar and talonavicular joints, without associated dislocation of the calcaneocuboid or tibiotalar joints, and without talar neck fracture. In 1853, Broca further classified these injuries into medial, lateral, and posterior, which refers to the direction that the foot takes in relation to the talus after the injury. This purely anatomic classification, which is widely used today, has prognostic value because of the functional outcomes associated with the different mechanisms.

Also referred to as basketball foot or acquired clubfoot, medial dislocations are the most common of subtalar joint dislocations, representing 80% of reported cases. The mechanism is usually that of high energy with forceful inversion of a plantarflexed foot. The injury is commonly associated with motor vehicle accidents as well as falls from a height.

The three articular facets of the subtalar joint are stabilized by the inherent bony structure as well as the capsuloligamentous supports. The dense talocalcaneal interosseous ligament is strengthened by the superficial deltoid medially and the calcaneofibular ligament laterally. For this injury to occur, all three of these ligaments must tear, sparing the calcaneonavicular "spring" ligament.

Clinically, the classic appearance is a medially displaced heel with severe inversion, plantarflexion, and adduction of the entire foot as well as apparent shortening of the medial border. Forty percent of cases involve an open injury; those that do not usually present with tenting over the dorsolateral aspect of the mid foot. Radiographically, the key element to accurate diagnosis is the relationship of the talar head to the navicular, which should be congruent on all views. In this injury, medial and plantar displacement of the navicular as well as medial displacement of the calcaneus, without disruption of the calaneocuboid joint, are also seen. Additionally, there often are associated fractures of the lateral navicular, dorsomedial talar head, posterior talar tubercle, and talar dome.

A prompt reduction is essential in avoiding skin necrosis and circulatory compromise. Reduction is easily achieved in the majority of patients by plantarflexion and inversion of the foot, followed by eversion and dorsiflexion. Applying direct pressure to the prominent talar head facilitates the reduction, which is often seen, heard, and felt. To assist reduction, the knee should be flexed to relax the pull of the gastrocnemius-soleus complex. Impediments to closed reduction include: buttonholing of the talar head through the extensor retinaculum, interposition of the deep peroneal neurovascular bundle. and impaction of the lateral navicular into the medial talar head. In these patients (5–10% of cases), open reduction is warranted. Post-reduction x-rays are important: the lack of deformity allows much better evaluation for associated fractures, especially talar dome injuries that significantly worsen the overall prognosis.

Overall outcomes vary inversely with the force of injury. Results are worse when intra-articular fractures are sustained, especially those involving the subtalar joint. Complications include skin necrosis, subtalar arthritis, instability, avascular necrosis, and infection.

In the present patient, the dislocation was reduced and maintained in cast immobilization.

Clinical Pearls

1. Medial subtalar joint (STJ) dislocations are high-energy injuries involving forceful inversion of a plantarflexed foot.

2. Forty percent of these injuries are open.

3. Medial STJ dislocation is often misinterpreted as an ankle dislocation.

4. Key diagnostic elements are talonavicular apposition and an intact calcaneal cuboid joint.

5. Associated fractures include: lateral navicular, dorsomedial talus, talar dome, and posterior talar process.

6. Post-reduction radiographs often uncover talar dome fractures.

7. Intra-articular fractures worsen the overall prognosis.

REFERENCES
1. Bellabarba C, Sanders R: Dislocations of the foot. In Surgery of the Foot and Ankle, 7th ed. St. Louis, Mosby Inc., 1999.
2. Bohay D, Manoli A: Subtalar joint dislocations. Foot Ankle Int 16(12):803–808, 1995.
3. Smith T: Dislocations. In Comprehensive Textbook of Foot Surgery, 2nd ed. Baltimore, Williams and Wilkins, 1992.

PATIENT 46

A 25-year-old runner with persistent ankle pain

A 25-year-old man presents with pain in his right ankle. He first experienced it while he was running with his son. Initially he thought that he may have sprained his ankle, but the pain still has not resolved after 3 months.

Physical Examination: Skin: right ankle moderately edematous, with loss of appearance of tendons compared to left foot and ankle; lateral aspect of right ankle warmer when compared to medial aspect. Musculoskeletal: pain elicited at distal aspect of fibula; ROM at ankle joint restricted due to pain and guarding; dorsiflexion, plantarflexion, inversion, and eversion all limited in comparison to contralateral joints.

Laboratory Findings: WBC, ESR: normal. Uric acid, creatinine clearance: normal. Radiographs: lytic lesion in distal fibula. MRI: expansile mass in metaphysis of distal right fibula, measuring $2 \times 2 \times 1$ cm; T1-weighted show soft tissue involvement with destruction of an adjacent cortical margin of bone; T2-weighted show increased signal intensity in distal fibula; mass well circumscribed; remaining osseous structures unaffected, with no change in signal intensity. Tc 99 bone scan: increased uptake on all three phases.

Course: Surgical pathology was performed and the results showed vascular channel hemorrhage and hemosiderin deposition. Multinucleated giant cells were also noted in the stroma.

Question: What is your diagnosis of this osseous lesion?

Diagnosis: Aneurysmal bone cyst

Discussion: In the presentation of aneurysmal bone cyst (ABC), the differential diagnosis should include osteosarcoma, giant cell tumor, chondroblastoma, and osteoblastoma. The clinical history of this patient is consistent with aneurysmal bone cyst for several reasons. First and foremost, a neoplastic lesion such as ABC should be considered in a patient who presents with pain and swelling for less than 3 months in the absence of trauma. Second, while aneurysmal bone cysts may be seen in any bone, they typically occur in the metaphysis of long bones, with an incidence of approximately 70%. Third, since 85% of aneurysmal bone cysts occur in patients under 20 years of age, an ABC must be considered in a younger patient.

Thorough evaluation of the radiographic features of aneurysmal bone cysts is crucial to narrowing the diagnosis. Radiographically, aneurysmal bone cysts may mimic malignant bone lesions due to their osteolytic, destructive nature and periosteal expansion. However, ABCs can be differentiated from more aggressive lesions by the classic eccentric blowout in the metaphysis of long bones in which the cortex remains intact. Each of these radiographic features was present in this patient's films, and all were further confirmed by MRI.

While the clinical presentation of this lesion certainly allows for inclusion of giant cell tumor in the differential diagnosis, the pathological and microscopic findings are more consistent with an ABC. Microscopically, ABCs exhibit blood-filled cavernous spaces separated by fibrous septae and the presence of multinucleated giant cells, as in this specimen. Intraoperatively, this lesion presented as a thin-walled space with copious amounts of blood. In addition to its clinical and radiographic presentation, the intraoperative appearance of an ABC along with the pathological findings confirm the diagnosis.

Despite being benign, aneurysmal bone cysts can be mistaken for malignant tumors both radiologically and pathologically due to their rapid growth rate and extensive osteolysis. ABCs are vascular anomalies, which are usually induced by minor or major trauma and may become associated with pathological fracture in approximately 20% of patients.

The treatment for these lesions consists of complete evacuation of the cavity with bone grafting. This is performed upon confirmation of the lesion's benign nature by frozen sectioning. If the joint is involved, arthrodesis is indicated in addition to the bone graft.

In the present patient, evacuation and bone grafting was successfully completed. He was immobilized for 6 weeks in a below-knee cast, received physical therapy for 2 weeks, and resumed normal activity within 2 months.

Clinical Pearls

1. When resecting the mass, care must be taken due to the thin nature of the cortical walls.

2. Inspection of nearby joints is important.

3. Due to their aggressive nature, aneurysmal bone cysts may be mistaken for malignant tumors. Clinical and radiographic presentations aid in the diagnosis, which is confirmed by pathological evaluation.

REFERENCES

1. Clough JR, Price CHG: Aneurysmal bone cysts: Review of 12 cases. J Bone Joint Surg (Br) 50:116, 1968.
2. Dahlin DC, McLeod RA: Aneurysmal bone cyst and other non-neoplastic conditions. Skel Radiol 8:243, 1982.
3. Koskinen EVS, Visuri TI, Holstrom T, Roukkula MA: Aneurysmal bone cyst. Evaluation of resection and of curettage in 20 cases. Clin Orthop Rel Res 118:136, 1976.
4. Kozlowski K, Middleton RWD: Aneurysmal bone cysts—Review of 10 cases. Aust Radiol 24:170, 1980.
5. Marberry K, Burd TA, Reddy R, Greene WB, Griffiths H: Intraosseus lipoma of the calcaneus. Orthopedics 24(3):225, 2001.
6. Resnick D, Niwayama G: Diagnosis of Bone and Joint Diseases, 2nd ed. Philadelphia, WB Saunders Company, 1988, pp 3730–3735, 3831–3842.

PATIENT 47

A 50-year-old woman with severe, recurring foot pain

A 50-year-old woman is experiencing pain in her left foot. She does not recall trauma to the area, but rather simply woke up one morning with the pain. After initial onset it continued for 6 weeks, but then gradually disappeared. It has now suddenly reappeared and is more severe, which prompted today's visit to the emergency department for evaluation. The patient relates that the pain seems to be most severe while she is ambulatory. She also mentions that she is unable to find any shoes that are comfortable. Previous medical history is significant for the removal of three basal cell masses from her face approximately 6 months earlier, and a mastectomy plus chemotherapy and radiation therapy about 2 years ago.

Physical Examination: General: healthy appearance. Musculoskeletal: pain in medial aspect of left foot. Skin: no edema, erythema, or calor. Gait: foot extremely painful on ambulation and in abducted position with obvious break in midtarsal region; antalgic gait; weight shift to lateral side of foot eases pain.

Laboratory Findings: Radiographs: expansile lytic area in first metatarsal base, occupying entire medullary region. Tc-99 scan: obvious uptake at base of first metatarsal in delayed phase; remainder of scan noncontributory for adjacent uptake. Pathology (from intraoperative biopsy): hyperchromatic, spindle-shaped cells separated by hyaline intercellular stroma.

Questions: What is the diagnosis of this lesion? What surgical option should be considered?

Diagnosis: Clear cell chondrosarcoma

Discussion: Clear cell chondrosarcomas occur more often in men than in women between the 3rd and 5th decades. These tumors are relatively common in the epiphyseal and metaphyseal regions of long tubular bones such as the femur and humerus, but they can occur in other bones. Reported to be slow growing, clear cell chondrosarcomas are often difficult to diagnose in bone because they are usually noted in the soft tissue. Clinical features include localized pain of long duration, limited motion at affected joints, and pathological fractures in 25% of patients.

Radiographically, these tumors are mostly osteolytic and slightly expansile, as in this case. For this reason, they must be differentiated from other tumors with similar radiographic presentations such as chondroblastoma, aneurysmal bone cyst, osteoblastoma, giant cell tumor, fibrosarcoma, osteosarcoma, and plasmacytoma. Additional radiologic signs may include endosteal erosions, soft tissue masses, and expansile margins that are sclerotic in nature.

Intraoperative evaluation reveals soft, granular cysts with clear or hemorrhagic fluid, as well as tumor cells with clear cytoplasm. Histologic confirmation of the lesion demonstrates compact cells in sheets with abundant clear cytoplasm and centrally located hyperchromic nuclei. Immune assay stains are an integral part of the diagnosis. Recurrence is high when conservative curettage is performed and therefore radical resection is both indicated and curative. Metastases to the brain, lungs, and other bones may occur.

The clinical and radiologic presentation of clear cell chondrosarcoma is quite similar to that of chondroblastoma. Due to the malignant nature of clear cell, these two entities must be differentiated. Clear cell chondrosarcoma can be distinguished based on its occurrence in an older patient population, and the presence of tumor cells upon examination. As with most neoplastic bone lesions, biopsy and pathological evaluation are critical to an accurate diagnosis.

In the present patient, the expansile lesion occupied the entire medullary region of the metatarsal, indicating that it had a high probability to metastasize. While potentially malignant, this lesion was advancing so slowly that it remained within the cortical margins of the metatarsal. Therefore, radical resection was required.

Clinical Pearls

1. If amputation is necessary, intraoperative biopsies to validate total resection are required at the amputation site.

2. Radiographic findings aid in narrowing the differential diagnosis of a clear cell chondrosarcoma based on tumor-specific features.

3. Bone biopsy remains the most accurate means of diagnosing clear cell chondrosarcoma.

REFERENCES

1. Bjornsson J, Unni KK, Dahlin DC, et al: Clear cell chondrosarcoma of bone. Observations in 47 cases. Am J Surg Pathol 8:223, 1984.
2. Gelczer RK, Wenger DE, Wold LE: Primary clear cell sarcoma of bone: A unique site of origin. Skel Radiol 28(4):240, 1999.
3. Kumar R, David R, Cierney G: Clear cell chondrosarcoma. Radiology 154:45, 1985.
4. Resnick D, Niwayama G: Diagnosis of Bone and Joint Disorders, 2nd ed. Philadelphia, WB Saunders Company, 1988, pp 3831–3842.
5. Volpe R, Mazabraud A, Thiery JP: Clear cell chondrosarcoma. Report of a new case and review of the literature. Pathologica 75:775, 1983.
6. Yokoyama R: Primary clear cell sarcoma of bone. Skel Radiol 29(5):302, 2000.

PATIENT 48

A 10-year-old boy with a limp

A 10-year-old boy presents with a 4-month history of limping. He has no history of trauma.

Physical Examination: Gait: obvious right foot drop. Musculoskeletal: limitation of dorsiflexion; strong power of plantarflexion. Vascular: dorsalis pedis and posterior tibial arteries palpable, with no trophic changes; no knee flexion or hip contractures; transmaleolar axis and hip rotation equal in external and internal motion. Neurologic: good sensation plantarly; dorsal decrease in two-point discrimination; deep tendon reflexes intact. Palpation: mass at proximal fibula; nontender, no redness.

Laboratory Findings: Radiographs: normal. MRI: 1-cm mass along fibular notch of fibula. EMG and nerve conduction velocities: decrease in velocities of peroneal nerve.

Question: What is your differential diagnosis?

Diagnosis: Ganglion with common peroneal nerve compression

Discussion: In the present patient, surgical removal and biopsy were performed. A ganglion was the most likely diagnosis, but neurilemmoma and neurofibroma had to be ruled out. Ganglions are common, and if they are located near a joint under the tight ligamentous bands covering nerves, entrapment can occur. This can be seen in the posterior and anterior tarsal tunnel. If proximally located, compression of the main nerve can lead to atrophy of the muscles innervated. In this patient, the ganglion was located in the lateral and anterior musculature. The result was an overpowering by the posterior group.

Due to ganglion locations, recurrence is still high after aspiration and injections with steroids. The motion at the joint level or tendon creates an irritation and produces a return of the hyaluronic acid.

Clinical Pearls

1. When a ganglion is located around a nerve, the ganglion needs to be followed completely to its origin. The stalk's origin is within a joint or tendon sheath. It must be removed completely or it will return.

2. Simple aspiration should be attempted first; however, it is usually unsuccessful, and the ganglion returns due to the local nature of the continual irritation at the site.

REFERENCES

1. Green DP, Hotchkiss R, Pederson WC (eds): Green's Operative Hand Surgery, 4th ed. New York, Churchill Livingstone, 1999.
2. McGlamry ED, et al : Comprehensive Textbook of Foot Surgery, 2nd ed. Baltimore, Williams & Wilkins, 1992, pp 1153–1154.
3. Stack RE: Compression of the common peroneal nerve by ganglion cysts. J Bone Joint Surg 47A(4):773–778. 1965.
4. Stedmans Medical Dictionary, 26th ed. Baltimore, Williams & Wilkins, 1995.

PATIENT 49

A 3-year-old boy with bowed legs

A 3-year-boy is referred for evaluation of increasing bowing of his legs. The mother and pediatrician state that the condition has progressively gotten worse since the child started walking when he was 9 months old. The child is quite healthy, and there are no other family members with bowing.

Physical Examination: General: significant bowing on frontal plane; transmaleolar axis 10° external bilaterally, with equal rotation of external and internal motion at knee joint. Gait analysis: no toe-in; no difficulty running or walking. Musculoskeletal: in knee flexion, dorsiflexion of foot at ankle 20°; in extension, 15°. Normal 2:1 ratio of inversion to eversion of subtalar joint; muscle function normal; knee joint stable, with no laxity or excessive motion.

Laboratory Findings: Radiographs (of knee): metaphyseal-diaphyseal angle 20°; metaphyseal beaking and thickening of medial cortices of tibiae bilaterally (see figure).

Questions: What condition is present? What are some of the causes of this bowing?

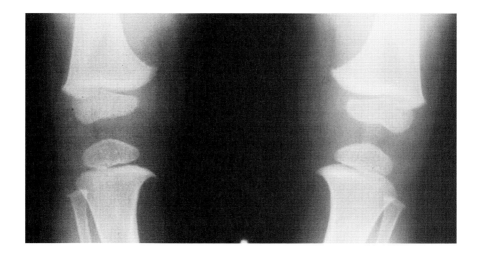

Diagnosis: Blount's disease (tibia vara)

Discussion: Infantile Blount's disease is progressive. The proximal tibia and the distal femur produce an abnormally high compressive force acting across the medial segment of the knee joint. This causes a retardation of growth in that area, or increased growth from the proximal aspect of the fibula and the lateral aspect of the proximal part of the tibia, or both. If a child begins walking at an early age, when the knees are still aligned in marked varus, then weight-bearing compressive forces will be greater on the medial aspect of the physis.

Continued compression results in limited growth of both the physis and the epiphysis. The medial aspect of the epiphysis becomes narrowed, and longitudinal growth from the medial aspect of the metaphysis is inhibited. Persistent internal tibial torsion also occurs. When children are not treated, severe degenerative joint disease develops during early adulthood.

Other causes of tibia vara include physiologic genu varum, which reduces as the child grows. Hypophosphatemic rickets—a sex-linked, dominant, inherited pattern—is the most common type of rickets creating a genu varum. The diagnosis is made after the child starts walking. Metaphyseal chondrodysplasia is an inherited disorder of bone growth that also causes bowing of the lower extremities. In the most common type of metaphyseal chondrodysplasia, height and limb alignment are within normal limits at birth, but genu varum persists, and retarded growth becomes obvious in the preschool years. Focal fibrocartilaginous dysplasia is an uncommon disorder that causes a unilateral and progressive tibia varum.

In the present patient with infantile tibia vara, an orthosis was prescribed. It was an above-the-knee brace with a free ankle, single medial upright, and no hinge joint at the knee. Every 6 weeks, the medial upright was bent to gain further valgus alignment at the knee.

Clinical Pearl

Indications for obtaining radiographs to differentiate tibia vara from physiologic bowing include:
- Genu varum that is relatively severe for the child's age
- Genu varum that has not improved or has gotten worse over the previous 3–4 months
- Excessive internal tibial torsion
- A positive family history for genu varum
- Marked asymmetry of limb alignment.

REFERENCES

1. Blount WP: Tibia vara. Osteochondrosis deformans tibiae. J Bone Joint Surg 19:1–29, 1937.
2. Drennan JC: Pediatric knee disorders. Instructional Course Lecture at the Annual Meeting of The American Academy of Orthopaedic Surgeons, Washington, D.C., Feb. 21, 1992.
3. Greene WB: Infantile tibia vara. Instructional Course Lectures, The American Academy Of Orthopaedic Surgeons. J Bone Joint Surg 75-A(1):130–143, 1993.
4. Greene WB, Kahler SG: Hypophosphatemic rickets: Still misdiagnosed and inadequately treated. Southern Med J 78: 1179–1184, 1985.
5. Langenskiold A: Tibia vara. A critical review. Clin Orthop 246: 195–207, 1989.

PATIENT 50

A 12-year-old boy with painful, aching ankles

A 12-year-old boy presents complaining of painful, aching ankles bilaterally. The pain is intermittent and of 4-week duration. It is aggravated occasionally by ambulation, but noted most markedly following periods of rest.

Physical Examination: General: multiple bony prominences at shoulders, elbows, wrists, fingers, knees, ankles, and hips. Orthopedic: mild lordosis of lumbar spine; 45° fixed forearm pronation bilaterally; 20° flexion contracture of hips, with 70° external and 20° internal rotation of femoral segment bilaterally; 1-cm limb length discrepancy, with right exceeding left; no pelvic tilt in stance; Allis sign positive; bilateral gastrocnemius-soleus equinus (left greater than right); mild tibial varum on left side; foot type with components of rearfoot and forefoot varus bilaterally. Musculoskeletal: rearfoot restricted frontal plane ROM bilaterally; hyperextended left hallux; adductovarus of 5th toe bilaterally; crepitus in both first metatarsophalangeal joints. Palpation: no pain over bony protuberances of medial malleolus nor at lateral ankle ligaments. Gait: toe-walking with no heel contact; posture was necessary for balance due to flexion contractures at hips and knees as well as sagittal plane spinal alignment.

Laboratory Findings: Radiographs (feet and ankles): multiple bilateral deformities consisting of shortened, stubby metatarsals and proximal phalanges; cystic areas in proximal phalanges; widened epiphyseal areas in bones of forefoot; grossly irregular epiphyses of lower legs, with widening of talotibial region—this area slanted on frontal plane bilaterally and gross bony overgrowths evident.

Question: What is your clinical diagnosis?

Diagnosis: Osteochondromatosis.

Discussion: Osteochondromatosis or osteo-cartilaginous exostoses are multiple protuberances from the surfaces of bones preformed in cartilage. Males are affected more frequently than females in a ratio of 3:1. It is an autosomal dominant finding, with exostoses on the metaphyseal regions of long tubular bones in a symmetrical fashion in children and adolescents. Malignant degeneration of multiple exostoses leading to chondrosarcomas is reported in less than 10% of cases.

The characteristic appearance of osteochondromatosis is the **trumpet sign:** a diffuse, club-shaped thickening of the metaphysis. The thickened area is usually covered by many sessile exostoses. In the lower extremity, both ends of the bones typically are involved; in the upper extremity, just one end of the tubular bone is involved. Interestingly, other than the calcaneus, all of the tarsal bones are spared of exostoses. Metatarsals are affected at any location of the shaft.

Osteochondromatosis is a benign condition of tumor-like masses at juxtaepiphyseal areas of long bones. In the lower extremity, the condition manifests itself as palpable bony masses near major joints, and these masses may restrict motion and compress neurovascular structures. Deformity of the metatarsals and phalanges is prominent in the foot. Ankle valgus and limb length discrepancy are additional noteworthy features. Surgical excision may be necessitated in cases of chronic pain or severe restriction of motion.

Secondary deformities arise due to shortening and angulation deformities. Rarely does the prominence cause direct pain unless there is soft-tissue swelling at the cartilaginous end of the exostosis. This fluid-filled bursae surrounds the exostosis. In the lower extremity, half of all the lesions are in the ankle; they are deformed with deviation or prominences.

The result of the deformities is compensation to the angular deviation. Treatment should address the compensation either by surgical or conservative realignment. If the bursa is painful, then the exostosis is removed. Multiple radiographic views may be needed to detect the presence of the exostosis in a child because the prominence may still be cartilaginous. An MRI may be indicated.

In the present patient, a biomechanical exam was performed, and orthotics were constructed to prevent frontal plane angular deviation.

Clinical Pearls

1. Always take multiple x-ray projections, as the exostosis may be sessile and therefore difficult to detect on a standard view.

2. MRIs are helpful in the young foot or with a prominence that is not seen radiographically. The outgrowth may be cartilaginous.

REFERENCES

1. Jahss M, Olives R: The foot and ankle in multiple hereditary exostoses. Foot Ankle 3:129, 1980.
2. Shapiro F, et al: Hereditary multiple exostoses. J Bone Joint Surg 61-A(6):816, 1979.

PATIENT 51

A 5-year-old boy with persistent left foot pain

A 5-year-old boy presents with a complaint of left foot pain that has been present for 2 months. The mother does not know of any trauma to the child's foot. This was his first experience with any type of pain.

Physical Examination: Palpation: pain on medial aspect of left foot. Skin: left foot mildly ruborous, with some increase in temperature as compared to right. Musculoskeletal: subtalar joint full and pain-free ROM; midtarsal joint normal ROM, but painful; pain localized to navicular area when first ray elevated.

Laboratory Findings: General: normal for age. Radiographs: increased radio-opacity; fragmented and narrow tarsal navicular bone; sclerosis; no pathology in remainder of osseous structures that were developed.

Questions: This child has which type of osteochondrosis? What are the appropriate treatments for this osteochondrosis?

Answers: Kohler's osteochondrosis. Appropriate treatments include rest, ice, and elevation; short leg cast; and orthotics.

Discussion: Kohler's osteochondrosis is more prevalent in boys than girls (4:1). Most of the time the disorder will resolve without treatment. However, reports indicate that immobilization decreases the symptoms and allows the condition to abate five times faster. This is usually a self-limiting disorder, and the navicular bone will reconstitute.

It is theorized that during the rapid growth phase of the single vessel supply of the tarsal navicular nucleus, disruption of this vessel could produce ischemia. This ischemia along with the forces of pronation and gravity cause fragmentation and collapse of the ossific nucleus, resulting in reactive hyperemia and pain. Kohler's disease is generally present in adolescent boys unilaterally and tends to spontaneously resolve over time. This osteochondrosis is thought to occur secondary to compression, similar to the way Freiberg's infraction of the second metatarsal head occurs.

Kohler's disease generally presents as pain and swelling along the medial midfoot of an active teenage male. The patient may be limping and unable to perform physical activity for any extended period of time secondary to discomfort. Evaluation reveals that pain increases upon weight bearing, and the child may supinate the foot to compensate for the pain on the medial side of the foot. Radiographs show an irregularly ossifying navicular bone with sclerosis, flattening, and possible fragmentation of the ossification center. The bone demonstrates an increased density of patchy areas. It also may appear uniformly dense. Magnetic resonance imaging reveals a homogenous decrease in signal intensity on T1-weighted images.

The initial treatment begins with rest, ice, and elevation of the affected foot. Limitation of the aggravating activity is often sufficient to calm the initial symptomotology. Several studies recommend short leg cast immobilization for approximately 2 months. The foot should be held in a plantarflexed and inverted position. Children casted for 2 months have complete resolution of pain and return to normal activity within 2.5 months. When the child is taken out of the cast it is recommended that an accommodative device be used for approximately 2 months. The medial side should be soft to limit pressure on the navicular. Permanent orthotics can be dispensed when the child is asymptomatic.

In the vast majority of patients, Kohler's disease eventually resolves without long-term sequelae. However, a distorted and sclerotic navicular bone may develop in some patients; this can lead to an arthritic talonavicular joint. If this is the case, a midtarsal joint arthrodesis may be required in adulthood.

The present patient was given a modified Cam walker, which consisted of a molded orthosis made of plastizoate. At the end of 3 weeks he was provided with a molded acrylic orthosis to prevent pronation.

Clinical Pearls

1. Midtarsal joint pain in a child whose bones have not completely ossified may be an indication of stress fracture. Though rare, the possibility should be considered—especially when there is no evidence of related trauma. Evaluate for the osteochondroses.

2. Bilateral films are most helpful in the diagnosis of Kohler's, as it is usually a unilateral deformity.

3. Pain is relieved by limiting the motion of the navicular bone.

REFERENCES
1. Ferguson AB, Gingrich RM: The normal and the abnormal calcaneal apophysis and tarsal navicular. Clin Orthop 10:87–95, 1957.
2. Waugh W: The ossification and vascularization of the tarsal navicular and their relation to Kohler's disease. J Bone Joint Surg 40-B:765–777, 1958.
3. Williams GA, Cowell HR: Kohler's disease of the tarsal navicular. Clin Orthop 158:53–58, 1981.

PATIENT 52

A 6-year-old girl with discomfort in her hands and feet

A 6-year-old girl is experiencing discomfort in her hands and feet. The pain is not related to any activity, as she has painful feet and ankles both after play and during rest. Her mother has noted daily temperature elevations and weight loss. The child's appetite has decreased, as well.

Physical Examinations: Musculoskeletal: range of motion of all joints normal. Palpation: tenderness of ankles and feet.

Watchful waiting was indicated, and the patient was sent home. Pain continued for a few months, gradually extending proximally to include all of her joints. On subsequent examination, the child's right ankle was red, hot, and swollen. Several lab tests were undertaken.

Laboratory Findings: Blood studies (from ankle): hemoglobin 10.5 g; white blood count 17,500/μl; 65 polymorphonuclear leukocytes, 29 lymphocytes, 6 eosinophils; ESR 34 mm/hr; latex fixation test negative; ASTO titer < 166 Todd units; febrile agglutinins normal; 5–7 white blood cells on urinalysis. Ankle aspirate: turbid fluid with a weak mucin clot. Radiographs (both feet): no changes in bone nor joints.

Question: An appropriate treatment for this child would be a daily regimen of what drugs?

Diagnosis: Juvenile rheumatoid arthritis

Discussion: About 70–80% of all adults with rheumatoid arthritis (RA) are positive for rheumatoid factor. In juvenile RA, the rate is 50%. If a child presents with rheumatoid factor, it is likely that juvenile RA will continue into adulthood. Juvenile RA symptoms disappear in more than half of all affected children.

Typically, the child looks ill and has high fevers and vague joint pain. Rashes, hepatosplenomegaly, lymphadenopathy, and leukocytosis usually develop. Also common is small stature, with resultant retardation of growth. Polyarthritis develops within the first few months and often is confused with septic joints.

Laboratory blood tests help rule out other conditions and classify the type of juvenile RA. ANA is found in the blood more often than rheumatoid factor, and both are found in only a small portion of juvenile RA patients. The rheumatoid factor test helps differentiate the three types of juvenile RA. Not all children with active joint inflammation have an elevated erythrocyte sedimentation rate.

Treatment options include:
- Nonsteroidal anti-inflammatory drugs (NSAIDs). These drugs often are the first type of medication used to treat juvenile RA. Most doctors do not treat children with aspirin because of the possibility that it will cause bleeding problems, stomach upset, liver problems, or Reye's syndrome. But for some children, aspirin in the correct dose (measured by blood test) can control juvenile RA symptoms effectively with few serious side effects.
- Disease-modifying anti-rheumatic drugs (DMARDs). If NSAIDs do not relieve symptoms, DMARDs slow the progression of juvenile RA. They often are taken with an NSAID because they take weeks or months to relieve symptoms. A variety of DMARDs are available, including hydroxychloroquine, oral and injectable gold, sulfasalazine, and d-penicillamine.
- Methotrexate. Researchers have learned that this type of DMARD is safe and effective for some children with RA whose symptoms are not relieved by other medications. Potentially dangerous side effects rarely occur because only small doses of methotrexate are needed to relieve arthritis symptoms. The most serious complication is liver damage, but it can be avoided with regular blood screening tests.
- Corticosteroids. These medications may be added to the treatment plan to control severe symptoms. They can be given either intravenously or orally.

Clinical Pearls

1. In adult rheumatoid arthritis, the disease is diagnosed by the presence or absence of rheumatoid factor (RF). RF is infrequently seen (less than 10%) in children.

2. When in doubt as to whether the diagnosis is septic joint or rheumatoid arthritis, a joint aspiration is indicated. Bacteriologic identification will establish the diagnosis of septic arthritis.

3. The main treatment of juvenile RA is to restore joint motion as soon as possible.

4. Therapeutic levels of salicylates can be achieved with a starting does of 60–80 mg per kilogram per day.

REFERENCES
1. Sharrard WJW: Paediatric Orthopaedics and Fractures. Blackwell Scientific, 1971.
2. Tachdijian MO: Pediatric Orthopaedics. Philadelphia, W.B. Saunders, 1972.

PATIENT 53

A 59-year-old man with a stiff hallux

A 59-year-old man presents with a chief complaint of pain in his right big toe for the past several months. The pain has become progressively worse in recent weeks. The toe is stiff, as well, and is most painful early in the morning when he first awakes. The patient relates no antecedent trauma to his big toe. The only treatment to date is over-the-counter ibuprofen, which was somewhat helpful for pain relief.

Past medical history includes non-insulin–dependent diabetes mellitus for 5 years and hypertension. Medications include Glucotrol XL 5 mg once a day and Lasix 20 mg twice a day. Allergies include sulfa drugs. Past surgical history is unremarkable. The patient does not smoke, and only uses alcohol socially.

Physical Examination: General: well nourished; no acute distress. Lower extremity: bilateral lower legs and feet; normal color, turgor, texture, and temperature. Pedal pulses: palpable bilaterally. Skin: mild erythema and minimal edema at first MCP joint of right foot; no open lesions. Musculoskeletal: mild tenderness at first MCP; considerable tenderness on ROM of first MCP, especially on extreme dorsiflexion; limited ROM on dorsiflexion, approximately 5°. Prominent area of bone palpable on dorsal aspect of first metatarsal head. Neurologic and manual muscle testing: normal bilaterally.

Laboratory Findings: Radiographs: lateral—large dorsal exostosis and arthritic changes within first MCP joint; anteroposterior (see figure)—head flattened, with loss of joint space; osteophytic changes noted along sides of joint; first ray elevated.

Question: What is the most likely cause of the patient's pain at the first MCP joint?

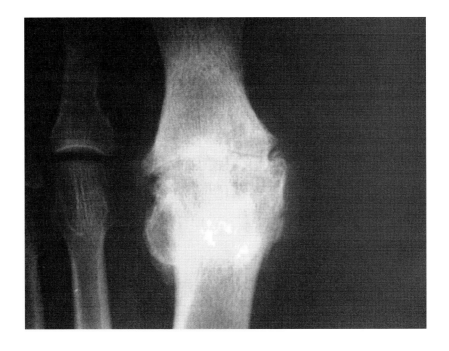

Diagnosis: Hallux limitus

Discussion: The patient has hallux limitus. On radiograph, significant joint space narrowing and some subchondral sclerosis are evident at the first MCP on the dorsal-plantar projection. The lateral projection reveals first metatarsal elevatus and some dorsal spurring, consistent with jamming at the joint, as well.

Hallux limitus is one of the most common entities encountered in a podiatric practice. It generally affects middle-aged patients, and is more prevalent in men than women. Some common etiologies include a long first metatarsal, metatarsus primus elevatus, trauma to the joint, and a hypermobile first ray. Each of these entities causes altered mechanics of the joint, resulting in the base of the proximal phalanx jamming against the head of the first metatarsal. Continuous jamming of the joint over time leads to changes within the joint as well as periarticularly.

These changes are generally visible on radiograph and are progressive in nature, with worsening joint signs and symptoms. Joint erosions cause narrowing of the joint, and jamming causes periarticular osteophyte formation, most notably along the dorsal aspect of the first metatarsal. The onset of the present patient's complaint coincides with the amount of joint destruction which has occurred to that point. As joint destruction continues, the patient compensates to decrease weight bearing at the first MCP joint. Compensatory complaints include lesser metatarsalgia, especially laterally, hyperflexion of the hallux IP joint causing shoe box pressure, and joint pain at the first metatarsal-cuneiform joint.

Conservative treatment includes altering the biomechanical abnormality contributing to the limited joint motion. For a first metatarsal elevatus, which is generally caused by a pes plano valgus deformity, initial therapy involves an orthotic insert with a first-ray cutout to allow plantarflexion of the metatarsal. For more advanced hallux limitus, an orthotic with a Morton's extension to limit first MCP joint motion can be helpful.

When patients fail to respond to conservative treatment, some type of surgical intervention may be required. Procedures to correct hallux limitus/rigidus can be classified into joint-sparing procedures and joint-destructive procedures. Joint-sparing procedures include simple cheilectomy to clean up periarticular osteophytes (see figure below), as well as metatarsal and hallucal osteotomies. If the level of joint adaptation is too great, then joint-destructive procedures can be done to restore pain-free range of motion at the first MCP. Destructive procedures include the Keller bunionectomy, joint replacement either with total or hemi-implant, and arthrodesis.

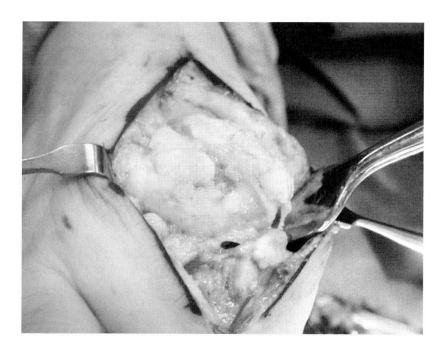

Clinical Pearls

1. The lateral radiographic projection is critically important. It will reveal a first ray elevatus, which caused the hypermobility that allowed the jamming of the great toe. The elevatus can be corrected if surgical intervention becomes necessary.

2. A stress dorsiflexion x-ray helps determine if an isolated dorsal condyle is present and will need to be removed. Jamming will continue, and if 10° of motion is attained on dorsiflexion, then consider a cheilectomy.

REFERENCES

1. Dannenberg HJ: Functional hallux limitus. J Am Pod Med Assoc 76:648–652, 1986.
2. Root M: Abnormal and Normal Function of the Foot. Los Angeles, Clinical Biomechanics Laboratory, 1977.

PATIENT 54

A 52-year-old woman with burning pain in her forefoot

A 52-year-old woman complains of an intermittent stabbing/burning pain in her right forefoot. The pain has progressively worsened over the last 6 months, and it is aggravated by her high-heeled shoes. She denies any preceding trauma to the area. Attempted treatment with ice and ibuprofen has been unsuccessful. Past medical history is significant for hypertension and gastroesophageal reflux disease (GERD), but the patient denies any previous back or foot injuries. She is taking Toprol XL and Prilosec. There are no known drug allergies. She is employed as a cosmetologist and is slightly overweight.

Physical Examination: General: no acute distress, well developed, well nourished, afebrile, vital signs stable. Neurologic: normal; sensation intact. Pedal pulses: palpable. Skin: mild right forefoot edema; no open lesions. Musculoskeletal: positive Tinel's sign; pain on compression of 3rd interspace. Gait: mild flexible pes planus foot type with adducto varus deformity to the 4th and 5th digits bilaterally. Manual muscle testing: grossly intact lower extremity muscles.

Question: What is your diagnosis?

Diagnosis: Morton's neuroma

Discussion: The condition we now refer to as Morton's neuroma was actually first described by an English chiropodist by the name of Durlacher in 1845. T.G. Morton of Philadelphia was given credit in 1876 following his description of a benign enlargement of the 3rd common digital branch off the medial plantar nerve located between the 3rd and 4th metatarsal heads. Today, we believe that this represents a mechanical entrapment neuropathy. It is most commonly found in the 3rd interspace of obese women who wear high-heeled, pointed shoes.

Patients typically present with complaints of discomfort from walking on a wrinkle in their stocking or feeling a lump in their shoe. The classic description is a "paroxysmal burning sensation," with an overwhelming desire to remove one's shoe. Only rarely is there a sensory deficit, and usually there is a degree of hyperesthesia. Clinically, patients will have pain (and often hear a click) when the involved web space is compressed between the thumb and index finger while the forefoot is squeezed. This has become known as a **positive Mulder's sign**. Additionally, patients may have radiating pain distally (Tinel's) or proximally (Valleix's).

The differential diagnosis includes metatarsal stress fractures, rheumatoid arthritis, Freiberg's infarction, bursitis, tarsal tunnel, peripheral neuropathy, and nerve root compression. While radiographs are useful to rule out other conditions, and MRIs can identify some neuromas, ultrasound is the most accurate diagnostic test. A normal interdigital nerve should be approximately 2 mm in diameter, and it usually becomes symptomatic when greater than 5 mm.

A Morton's neuroma is actually not a neuroma, and it is not a neoplasm. It is a tumorous nodule (see figure) formed by hyperplasia of both axons and Schwann cells. The degenerative process that occurs is characterized by endoneural and neural edema; perineural, epineural, and endoneural fibrosis; and hypertrophy.

Conservative care includes wider shoes, arch supports, metatarsal pads ("met cookies"), low dye strapping, and custom-molded orthotics. The goal of biomechanical adjustment is to limit pronatory hypermobility. Other methods include injections with steroid or dilute 4% alcohol (sclerosing). Historically, conservative treatment provides symptomatic relief in 20–30% of cases.

When conservative treatment fails, surgical excision has a 76–96% success rate. The most common approach is dorsal longitudinal incision, as described by Mckeever in 1952. Careful dissection and meticulous hemostasis are extremely important, as is a clean transection of the nerve to prevent postoperative hematomas, and recurrent stump neuromas.

In the present patient, nonsurgical means failed to relieve the condition. Therefore, she underwent surgical excision. A dorsal curvilinear incision was made over the third interspace, exposing the neuroma, which was then dissected free and removed. Postoperative assessment at 6 months revealed a healed incision site and no recurrence of pain.

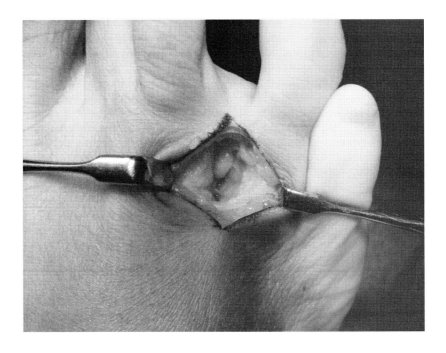

Clinical Pearls

1. Morton's neuroma is an entrapment neuropathy. The typical patient is an overweight female in high-heeled shoes
2. Patients complain of a paroxysmal burning sensation.
3. Mulder's sign is an important diagnostic aid.
4. Ultrasonagraphy is the most convenient, most accurate, and least expensive diagnostic test.
5. Histopathology is consistent with perineural fibrosis.
6. Neuromas are always located distal to the metatarsal heads.

REFERENCES

1. Miller S: Morton's neuroma: A syndrome. In McGlamry ED, Banks AS, Downey MS (eds): Comprehensive Textbook of Foot Surgery, 2nd ed. Baltimore, Williams and Wilkins, 1992.
2. Wu K: Morton's interdigital neuroma: A clinical review of its etiology, treatment, and results. J Foot Ankle Surg 35(2): 112–119, 1996.

PATIENT 55

A 40-year-old man with a progressively flattened foot after a minor fall

A 40-year-old man presented to the emergency department (ED) after falling off a stool and injuring his left foot. Physical examination at that time revealed edema and a superficial abrasion on the dorsomedial aspect of the left foot. The patient exhibited pain on palpation of the medial metatarsal area; the pain was exacerbated by weight-bearing and ambulation. Pertinent medical history was significant only for a long history of insulin-dependent diabetes mellitus. Medical management of his diabetes included 60 units of Humulin insulin in the morning and 40 units in the evening. The patient related that he was allergic to Keflex and Neomycin. Vital signs were stable, and the neurovascular status was intact to both feet.

At that time, x-rays were negative for fracture and dislocation, and the patient was diagnosed as having a sprain of his left foot. Treatment consisted of cleansing the superficial abrasion and dispensing a 4-inch ACE bandage. Instructions were for RICE therapy, weight-bearing as tolerated, and follow-up with his local medical doctor.

One week later, the patient returned to the ED complaining of persistent pain and swelling. Upon physical examination he stated that he had reinjured the same foot earlier that day and felt "bones move" in his foot. The left foot was remarkable for edema and ecchymosis dorsally, with pain on palpation of the medial plantar longitudinal arch. The abrasion was healing, and there were no signs of infection. Neurovascular status remained intact to both feet. Another set of foot radiographs was obtained and compared to the previous films, which revealed no change. Again, a diagnosis of sprain/strain to the left foot was made. The patient was instructed to remain non-weight-bearing on the left foot and was given an appointment to follow-up with the orthopedics department. The orthopedist casted the limb for 6 weeks non-weight-bearing.

Ten months later the patient returned with a deformation of his left foot involving a prominent bump and marked build-up of callus on the plantar aspect. The patient was weight-bearing in an ankle-foot orthosis, but complained of pain by the end of the day and an inability to ambulate comfortably.

Physical Examination: Skin: swelling, erythema. Temperature: increased from midfoot to tarsometatarsal area. Neurovascular: status intact; however, diminished sharp-dull response. Pedal pulses: strong and bilaterally symmetrical. Gait: forefoot abducted upon rearfoot, with depression of medial longitudinal arch. Musculoskeletal: large, medial, bony protuberance.

Laboratory Findings: Radiographs (new): marked destruction at Lisfranc's articulation fragmentation, including disintegration and osteolysis; medial cuneiform dislocated from medial column (see figures). Technetium 99 and Indium 111 studies: both positive, so infection could not be ruled out. Culture and sensitivity: negative. Gram stain: negative. Pathology: benign bone with fibrous marrow, increased osteoblastic activity, few mononuclear inflammatory cells, and surrounding dense fibrous tissue; no evidence of osteomyelitis.

Question: What disease state needs to be ruled out?

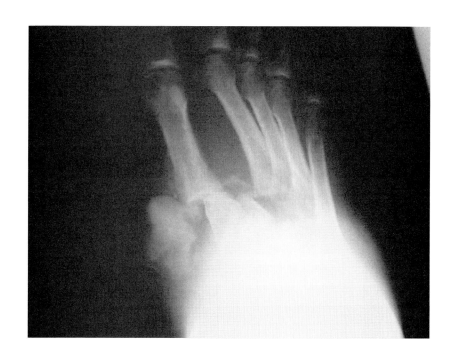

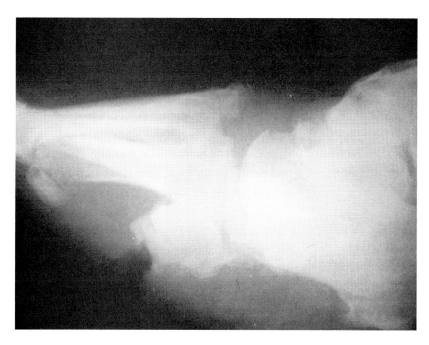

119

Diagnosis: Charcot joint

Discussion: Lisfranc's joint is the usual location of Charcot breakdown in a patient that is not excessively pronated and has a stable midtarsal joint. Patients that are pathologically pronated in stance tend to suffer breakdown within and around Chopart's joint. The breakdown can start with an episode of macrotrauma or repetitive microtrauma across the joints. A primary or secondary contracture of the tendo-achilles, which limits the dorsiflexion of the foot on the ankle, is usually seen. Since dorsiflexion cannot occur at the ankle, the midtarsal joint starts to dorsiflex. This is the microtrauma that occurs within the diabetic patient, and the entire foot starts to pronate and collapse.

The clinical appearance of the Charcot foot involves dorsiflexion and abduction at Lisfranc's or Chopart's joints. The dorsiflexion component originates from the stress of push off during ambulation, and is exaggerated in the patient who is extremely pronated in stance. A distinct pathophysiologic characteristic in Charcot is destruction of the plantar ligaments and atrophy of the plantar intrinsic musculature. This means that the Windlass action of Hicks is not functioning properly, and the plantar tension banding effect which produces stability within the tarsal joints is not present. The loss of this important stabilizing mechanism encourages ground reactive forces to dorsiflex the forefoot during propulsion.

One notable point in regard to Lisfranc's breakdown is the abduction of the forefoot on the rearfoot. This author believes that the pull of the peroneus longus and peroneus brevis is mainly responsible for the abduction. Once the breakdown begins, the first ray assumes a dorsiflexed position, and the action of the peroneus longus changes from plantarflexion and eversion to abduction.

Although the peroneus longus is responsible for some of the abduction in the Charcot foot, it is the pull of the peroneus brevis that provides the main abduction force. The peroneus brevis inserts distal to the breakdown and is unopposed in its abduction pull. The tibialis anterior also has its insertion distal to the Lisfranc breakdown, but has little abductory force at this level to oppose the peroneus brevis. The tibialis posterior has some slips that insert distal to the breakdown, but largely it inserts into the navicular and acts as a stabilizer of the midtarsal joint. Therefore, the continuous unopposed pull of the peroneus longus and peroneus brevis muscles is the main deforming force responsible for the abduction of the forefoot on the rearfoot, in the patient with a Charcot breakdown at Lisfranc's joint.

The pathogenesis of the neuropathic joint has been debated since it was first described. It is believed to be a combination of several factors: (1) the loss of neurologic protective mechanisms, (2) osteolysis/demineralization secondary to autonomic neuropathy, and (3) stress applied to the weakened bone surrounding joints, producing fractures and initiating the Charcot process.

In the present patient, conservative control by immobilization to allow the active stage to reduce was successful for a short period. Long-term immobilization was undertaken via a medial column fusion, and the patient was given an orthosis postoperatively.

Clinical Pearls

1. The initial concern—regardless of treatment—must be to rule out osteomyelitis.

2. It is imperative to allow the acute-phase Charcot joint to calm down, to prevent further damage to the involved joints.

3. Realignment of soft and osseous tissue prevents further breakdown.

4. Realignment of the forefoot-to-rearfoot relationship decreases the possibility of a return of Charcot changes.

REFERENCES

1. Banks AS, McGlamry ED: Diabetic and Diabetic Charcot Foot Reconstruction. Reconstruction Surgery of the Foot and Leg, Update 89. Atlanta, GA, Podiatry Institute, 1989.
2. Lesko P: Talonavicular dislocations and midfoot arthropathy on neuropathic diabetic foot. Clin Orthop 240:226,1989.

PATIENT 56

A 14-year-old boy with persistent pain in his knee

A 14-year-old boy presents with pain in his right knee. He has been experiencing the pain for 3 months, and it has not improved with rest or elevation. He plays basketball every afternoon, and when the game is completed the pain is excruciating. He does not remember injuring this knee and denies any history of high fevers this past year.

Physical Examination: Palpation: proximal aspect of right leg swollen and quite tender. Musculoskeletal: knee joint normal ROM compared to opposite side; no pain on motion; active extension of right leg difficult, with tightness in hamstrings; full extension could not be maintained when leg actively flexed; McMurray and Lachman tests and patella tracking negative.

Laboratory Findings: Radiographs: soft tissue swelling anterior to the tibial tuberosity, with fragmentation of tibial tubercle (see figure). MRI: increased signal in infrapatellar bursa.

Question: What disease is affecting this apophysis?

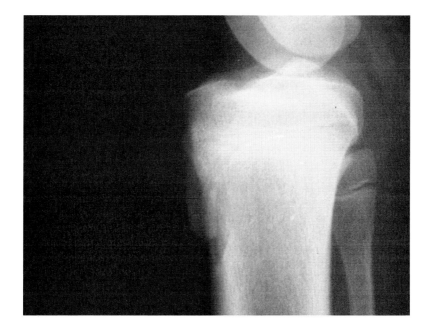

Diagnosis: Osgood-Schlatter disease

Discussion: A common condition of Osgood-Schlatter's disease is an apophysitis of the tibial tuberosity. It is believed to be the result of microavulsions caused by repeated traction on the anterior portion of the developing ossification center of the tibial tuberosity. Inflammation and reparative changes cause pain, swelling, and tenderness.

Osgood-Schlatter's is referred to as osteochondrosis, but avascular necrosis seems unlikely since the blood supply in the present patient is excellent. It is an overuse syndrome that occurs between 9 and 15 years of age. Osgood-Schlatter's affects the adolescent apophysis of the proximal tibia (particularly in young athletes) and is more commonly seen in boys than girls (3:1) There is a frequent history of repetitive running and jumping that initiates the process. Pain and swelling over the tibial tubercle is diagnostic of the disease. The characteristic physical finding is a "knobby knee." There may be erythema surrounding the swollen tibial tubercle.

X-rays can be confirmatory, but seldom diagnostic. All children of this age group usually have fragmentation on x-ray of the tibial tuberosity. The fragments occasionally do not unite, causing a separate ossicle to remain into adulthood. These ossicles may be symptomatic, requiring removal.

In the present patient, treatment consisted of rest and removal from strenuous activity. A cylinder cast was placed from the ankle to the thigh in extension.

Clinical Pearls

1. Conservative treatment for apophysitis is paramount, because 90% of cases resolve even with rest as the only treatment.

2. Never instill any type of steroid in this disorder: steroids are contraindicated.

3. Always maintain the strength of the patellar tendon, but do not over stress the tendon. The child should refrain from all rigorous activity.

REFERENCES
1. Krause BL, et al: Natural history of Osgood-Schlatter's disease. J Pediatr Orthop 10:65, 1990.
2. Kujala UM, et al: Osgood-Schlatter's disease in adolescent athletes. Am J Sports Med 13(4):236, 1985.
3. Ogden JA, et al: Osgood-Schlatter's disease and tibial tuberosity development. Clin Orthop 116:180, 1976.

PATIENT 57

A 27-month-old girl who is unable to walk

A 27-month-old girl is evaluated for an inability to walk. The child just arrived from an eastern European country after being adopted by an American couple. Very little prenatal history is available, other than that the child was premature. The exact gestational age is unknown.

Physical Examination: General: lower 10% for height and weight. Gait: not walking. Musculoskeletal: delayed motor functions; legs severely bowed (see figure). Neurologic: delayed mental functions.

Laboratory Findings: Radiographs: rachitic changes of distal femoral epiphyseal line; epiphysis widened; severe angular bowing of tibia evident on frontal and saggital planes. Alkaline phosphotase: mildly increased.

Question: What vitamin deficiency is present in this child?

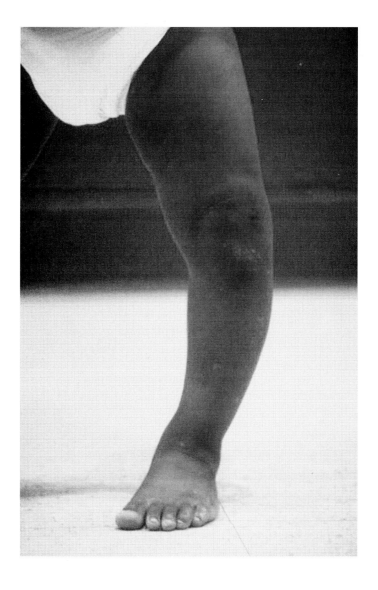

Diagnosis: Vitamin D is deficient.

Discussion: Children with dietary rickets (simple vitamin-resistant rickets) are normally seen between 6 months and 3 years of age. Incidence of dietary rickets increases with prematurity. Rickets involves insufficient intake of vitamin D and inadequate exposure to sunlight. It is a very rare finding in the United States. Children who are on anticonvulsive medications have to be observed for simple dietary rickets.

The clinical features of dietary rickets are muscular weakness and lethargy. The present patient has a protuberant abdomen. Walking and standing are usually delayed because structural support is insufficient; the child will experience stress fractures in and about the metaphyseal-epiphyseal junctions. The smooth metaphyseal-epiphyseal junction is distorted and bulbous because of the failure of the orderly endochondral bone sequence. Additionally, the ankles, knees, and wrists are thickened.

The treatment of vitamin D–deficient rickets is simple vitamin D, which can be obtained in fortified milk. The recommended dosage is 2000 to 5000 international units for 6–12 weeks. If this fails, the problem is not vitamin-sensitive rickets, but renal tubular insufficiency or renal refractory rickets.

In the present patient with dietary rickets, simple treatment with fortified vitamin D milk reversed the process.

Clinical Pearls

1. Bowing of the legs is the characteristic finding in rickets.
2. The diagnosis is predominately made by metabolic and clinical changes.
3. Radiographic findings vary in rickets and are not reliable for diagnosis.
4. In all forms of rickets, therapy must be started first before consideration of bracing or surgery to correct the structural problems.

REFERENCE
Oestreich AE: Skeletal System, Practical Pediatric Imaging. Diagnostic Radiology of Infants and Children, 2nd ed. Boston, Little, Brown, 1991, pp 263–410.

PATIENT 58

A 12-year-old boy with a painful and swollen ankle

A 12-year-old boy presents with a history of pain and swelling of his right ankle. The pain first began when he returned to school after his summer vacation in New England. He has no history of trauma, other than a "normal" ache he feels in his ankle after he runs. His mother noticed that the ankle would occasionally be red and swollen, and it did not respond to nonsteroidal anti-inflammatory drugs (NSAIDs), ice, or elevation. The child has no history of fevers, chills, or rashes.

Physical Examination: General: ankle moderately swollen; no local swelling in groin or popliteal areas; no other joint swelling or pain. Gait: antalgic. Musculoskeletal: ROM of ankle limited in dorsiflexion/plantarflexion as well as inversion/eversion. He had

Laboratory Findings: Radiographs (right ankle): increased soft tissue swelling, consistent with joint effusion; no bony abnormalities. Aspiration: fluid straw-colored. ELISA titre for Lyme disease: 1:640. Western blot: positive.

Questions: What is the diagnosis? What is the relevance of the serologic testing?

Diagnosis: Lyme disease

Discussion: This is a multisystem infection caused by the spirochete, *Borrelia burgdorferi,* and transmitted by the Ixodes deer tick. The late, persistent infection (stage 3) of Lyme arthritis is quite common in children. Characteristically, it is monoarticular and usually affects the larger joints. The joint effusion typically is increased and not consistent with the amount of pain.

ELISA is the test most commonly employed in the diagnosis of Lyme disease. The study detects the antibodies (IgG and IgM) of the spirochete and is very sensitive in the later stage of arthritic involvement. It is not sensitive in the early stages, with an increase in false positives; for this reason a Western blot is used to confirm.

In the present patient, intra-articular steroids and NSAIDs were given to lessen the articular inflammatory response. The patient was placed on doxycycline 100 mg BID for 30 days, and an EKG was obtained to rule out cardiac abnormalities.

Clinical Pearls

1. Children are less likely to develop chronic Lyme arthritis with associated joint destruction.

2. The differential diagnosis should include septic arthritis, juvenile rheumatoid arthritis, and reactive arthritis (e.g., toxic synovitis, Reiter's syndrome).

3. Severity of joint effusion and pain can wax and wane for several months. When there is a history of joint pain and no trauma, rule out Lyme disease with serologic testing.

REFERENCES
1. Evans J: Lyme disease. Curr Opin Rheumatol 7(4):322–328, 1995.
2. Jouben LM, Steele RJ, Bono JV: Orthopaedic manifestations of Lyme disease. Orthop Rev 23(5):395–400, 1994.
3. Kalish R: Lyme disease. Rheum Dis Clin North Am 19(2):399–426, 1993.
4. Lawrence SJ: Lyme disease: An orthopaedic perspective. Orthop 15(11):1331–1335, 1993.

PATIENT 59

A 17-year-old boy with a red, swollen toe

A 17-year-old boy presents with redness and swelling of the lateral nail border of his hallux. These symptoms arose about 1 month ago. He has a history of multiple infections of this hallux border, and his primary care physician has prescribed multiple courses of antibiotic therapy. The patient's hallux would improve during the course of treatment, but would flare up again after a few weeks.

Physical Examination: Temperature 97.9° F; pulse 62; respirations 15; blood pressure 98/69. Skin: erythematous, edematous hallux lateral border with sloughing at periphery of erythema; otherwise normal. HEENT: normal. Chest: clear. Cardiac: normal. Abdomen: nontender. Lower extremity: palpable DP and PT pulses; diffuse tenderness, proud flesh, erythema, edema, and purulent drainage on hallux medial nail border (see figure).

Laboratory Findings: WBC 5000/µl; Hg 16.7; Hct 36.9; platelets 300,000/µl. Urinalysis: normal.

Question: What is the diagnosis?

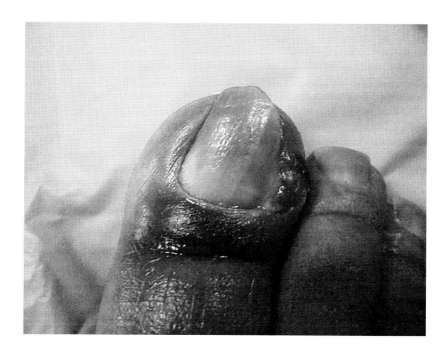

Diagnosis: Ingrown toenail with secondary bacterial infection

Discussion: Paronychia is defined as inflammation of nail borders. The inflammation is caused by a portion of the nail implanting itself into the soft tissues of the nail border as the nail grows. The offending portion may arise from improper trimming of the nails or from trauma. This spicule of nail causes a foreign body reaction and an inflammatory response, and the area can become secondarily infected by bacteria.

The bacteria that invade the area usually infect the surrounding tissue rather than the nail plate. The most common organisms isolated from infected surrounding tissues are Staphylococcus, Streptococcus, *Escherichia coli,* Pseudomonas, and Proteus. Pseudomonas is capable of infecting the nail plate and causing a blue-green discoloration called a pyocyanin.

When evaluating a patient with an apparent paronychia it is important to rule out other entities. X-rays should be taken to aid in diagnosis. Osteomyelitis can occur from a puncture wound, chronic paronychia, or ulceration, and can present as a simple paronychia that waxes and wanes with antibiotic therapy. Subungal exostosis can also mimic a recurrent paronychia secondary to pressure abnormalities; it should be treated appropriately with surgical excision or increased-depth shoes. Both benign and malignant neoplasms are often mistaken for paronychias. Some common tumors that can be misdiagnosed are osteochondroma, melanoma, squamous cell carcinoma, verruca, acquired digital fibrokeratoma, periungal fibroma, myxoid cyst, and pyogenic granuloma.

Clinical examination and history are very important in making the proper diagnosis. Laboratory studies are usually not indicated because systemic involvement is rare. Culture and sensitivities should be taken if drainage is present; however, most paronychias clear before culture results are returned. If tumor is suspected, a biopsy should be performed.

The gold standard for treatment of a paronychia is to remove the offending border of nail. Until this portion of the nail is removed, the problem will not resolve. Antibiotics should be initiated if the patient has systemic involvement or extensive cellulitis, or is immunocompromised. If hypertrophic flesh is present, excision or silver nitrate can be used to remove granulation tissue. Some suggest that a V cut into the distal tip of the nail can be used to relieve pressure in the corners, but this author has not seen success with this treatment.

Clinical Pearls

1. Paronychia can develop from improper nail clipping, trauma from excessive pronation, or improper shoe gear.
2. Other etiologies must be ruled out by x-ray or biopsy.
3. The gold standard of treatment is to remove the offending nail spicule.
4. Antibiotics are not necessary except in cases of extensive cellulitis, immune system compromise, nonresponse to previous therapy, or systemic involvement.

REFERENCES
1. Berlin SJ: A laboratory review of 67,000 foot tumors and lesions. J Am Pod Assoc 74:341–347, 1984.
2. Gunnoe RE: Disease of the nails: How to recognize and treat them. Postgrad Med 74:357–362, 1983.

PATIENT 60

A 41-year-old woman with a darkened and painful toe

A 41-year-old woman presents with pain in the distal aspect of her right second toe for several days. She is secondarily concerned about darkening and discoloration of the digit at the medial aspect of the proximal nail fold. The patient denies any trauma to the area. Symptoms are not aggravated by walking, weight bearing, or any particular shoe gear. However, she does relate that her current complaint seems to correspond to the change in the weather and is particularly symptomatic with cold weather. She has received no treatment for this condition. Previously, a partial second-digit amputation was performed on the patient's left foot, and multiple digital amputations were performed on her bilateral hands.

Physical Examination: HEENT: normal. Chest: clear. Cardiac: regular. Abdomen: nontender. *Lower extremity*—Pulses: dorsalis pedis and posterior tibial 2/4 bilaterally. Vascular: immediate capillary refill to digits. Temperature gradient: normal proximal to distal cooling of leg to digits. Skin: no ecchymosis or edema of right second digit or foot; mild darkening/ discoloration of distal aspect of right second digit, but no gangrene; healed left 2nd digit incision site. Neurologic: epicritic sensation intact. Musculoskeletal: motor function of lower extremity/foot intact, no orthopedic deformity. *Upper extremity*—Partial amputation of digits 2, 4, and 5 of right hand, and of thumb and digits 2–5 of left hand at proximal and distal interphalangeal joints.

Laboratory Findings: CBC with diffential: normal. Chemistry profile: normal. Radiographs: *Right foot*—partial second-digit amputation; no bony regrowth at remaining portion of proximal phalanx; mild diffuse osteopenia; no vascular calcifications. *Left foot*—Mild diffuse osteopenia, no osseous pathology of 2nd digit or foot; no vascular calcification; joint space of 2nd interphalangeal joints congruous and without contracture or deformity.

Question: What is cause of the patient's symptoms in her right second digit and the multiple digital amputations?

Diagnosis: Raynaud's disease

Discussion: Raynaud's disease is an idiopathic, symmetrical, and bilateral contraction or spasm of the small arteries or arterioles of the digits of the hand and the foot. The etiology seems to be an extreme sensitivity to cold temperatures. An attack can also occur as a result of an emotional response or event, although this is rare. The primary treatment for the attack or condition is warming of the extremity.

The diagnosis of Raynaud's is made from the patient's history—particularly the response to temperature changes—and physical examination. The clinician must keep in mind a few key points when considering Raynaud's as a disease entity, or cause of local gangrene or infection to a digit. The disease is more prevalent in females; it primarily affects those aged 14–40; and it usually involves both the hands and the feet. Examine both the upper and lower extremities, and look for color changes in the digits. The color changes can go from white to blue to red, depending on the stage of the attack, and are typically accompanied by pain.

If gangrene or infection sets in as a result of the disease, it must be treated accordingly. A local soft-tissue infection may be treated with debridement and antibiotics. A partial or complete digital amputation may be necessary to properly treat gangrene or osteomyelitis.

The present patient had immediately warmed her extremity when she felt the onset of symptoms, and as a result her attack was reversible. The pain in her second digit was slowly resolving, and the color change was most likely related to previous attacks. Gangrene did not set in; therefore, surgical intervention and/or amputation was not necessary. The patient was reminded of the need to avoid cold water and cold temperatures to prevent another attack or further amputation.

Clinical Pearls

1. Digital pressures in a patient with Raynaud's disease may be normal or diminished depending on the temperature of the room when the noninvasive vascular test is performed.

2. Gangrene of a digit may occur in the presence of normal arterial pulses.

3. Raynaud's affects the digits of the hand more commonly than the feet, and the involvement is usually bilateral and symmetrical.

4. Raynaud's primarily occurs because of a local sensitivity of the digital vessels to cold. Rarely, it can occur as a result of emotional arousal.

5. Pallor (white), cyanosis (blue), and reactive hyperemia (red) are the typical colors seen in the digits upon an acute Raynaud's attack and subsequent resolution or rewarming of the extremity.

REFERENCE

Creager MA, Dzau VJ: Vascular diseases of the extremities. In Isselbacher K, Braunwald E, Wilson J, et al (eds): Harrison's Principles of Internal Medicine, 13th ed. New York, McGraw-Hill, Inc., 1994, pp 1135–1143.

PATIENT 61

An 86-year-old man with chronic foot pain

An 86-year-old man presented with a 6-month history of right foot pain. Pain was present only with weight bearing, causing him to discontinue walking. Previously he had walked 2.5 miles daily. His past history was remarkable only for hypertension treated with a diuretic. He had undergone bunionectomy of the left foot but denied trauma to the right foot.

Physical examination: Temperature 97.8°, pulse 80, respirations 18, blood pressure 160/90. Skin: normal. Lymph nodes: normal. HEENT: atherosclerotic retinal vasculature. Neck: no bruit. Chest: clear. Heart: normal. Abdomen: normal. Neurologic: decreased sensation to light touch, pinprick and thermal sensation below the knees, markedly decreased joint position sense in the toes, normal in the fingers, absent ankle jerks. Musculoskeletal: warmth and swelling over dorsum of right midfoot with collapsed plantar arch and normal ankle motion.

Laboratory findings: WBC 8,000/μL; Hct 41.5%; platelets 249,000/μL; Na$^+$ 140 mmol/L; K$^+$ 3.5 mmol/L; Cl$^-$ 98 mmol/L; CO$_2$ 32 mmol/L; BUN 28 mg/dL; glucose 139 mg/dL; creatinine 1.3 mg/dL; calcium 9.6 mg/dL. Synovial fluid analysis: yellow, cloudy; WBC 11 cells/μL with 33% neutrophils, 7% lymphocytes, 60% macrophages; glucose 90 mg/dL; urate and CPPD crystals absent. STS: negative. Foot radiograph: healed fractures at midshaft of 2nd and 3rd metatarsals with evidence of old Lisfranc's fracture and osteoarthritic changes involving the tarsal bones. Technetium-MDP bone scan (shown below): increased activity on flow, immediate and delayed images of right foot.

Question: What is the diagnosis?

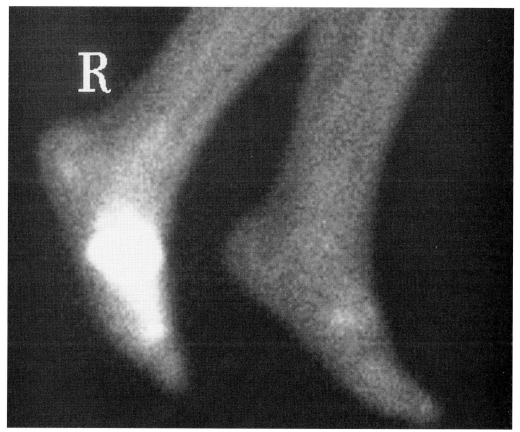

Diagnosis: Diabetic neuroarthropathy (Charcot joint).

Discussion: Charcot described the association of certain arthropathies with neurologic diseases—primarily tabes dorsalis—and the term "Charcot joint" is now applied to most articular abnormalities related to neurologic deficits. The terms neuroarthropathy and neutrophic and neuropathic joint disease are synonymous with Charcot joint. Neuropathy leads to loss of protective sensations of pain and proprioception which, in turn, lead to recurrent joint injury, malalignment, and progressive degeneration of the articulation.

Lesions of the central or peripheral nervous systems can lead to neuroarthropathy. Examples include syphilis (tabes dorsalis), syringomyelia, meningomyelocele, traumatic spine lesions, Charcot-Marie-Tooth disease, diabetes mellitus, alcoholism, pernicious anemia, and intra-articular administration of steroids. The distribution of the articular involvement varies among the neurologic disorders and may be a clue to diagnosis. Tabes dorsalis, complicated by neuroarthropathy in 5 to 10% cases, most commonly involves the knee, hip, ankle, or spine. Syringomyelia affects the shoulder, elbow, wrist, or spine. Alcoholism affects the foot and toes.

Diabetes mellitus is now a more frequent cause of neuroarthropathy than is syphilis. Neuroarthropathy has been noted in 0.15% of hospitalized diabetic patients, but the true incidence may be greater. Typically, diabetic neuroarthropathy occurs in the patient with long-standing diabetes mellitus. Occasionally, as in the present case, neuroarthropathy may be the initial clinical manifestation of diabetes mellitus. The joints in the forefoot and midfoot are most commonly affected, although the ankle, knee, spine, and joints of the upper extremities also can be affected. Osseous fragmentation, sclerosis and subluxation or dislocation occur in the intertarsal or tarsometatarsal joints. The radiographic findings in the foot may resemble an acute Lisfranc's fracture-dislocation in which fracture at the base of the metatarsals (2nd–5th) and cuboid is associated with lateral dislocation of the 2nd through 5th metatarsal bones. Scintigraphy with bone-seeking radionuclides shows areas of increased accumulation of the radionuclide.

Bony eburnation, fracture, subluxation, and joint disorganization are more profound in neuroarthropathy than in any other arthropathy. Early cases may resemble osteoarthritis. Calcium pyrophosphate dihydrate crystal deposition (CPPD) disease can resemble neuroarthropathy, or may coexist with neuroarthropathy. Similar destructive changes may occur in the shoulder with calcium hydroxyapatite crystal deposition. Osteomyelitis, particularly in the diabetic foot, may mimic or be superimposed on a neuroarthropathy. An [111]indium-labeled white blood cell scan may help differentiate infected from noninfected rapidly progressive neuroarthropathy.

Treatment includes discerning the underlying cause of neuropathy. Diabetic neuroarthropathy of the foot may respond to a total-contact cast or brace. Some cases improve with arthrodesis; those that fail may require amputation.

In the present case, a diagnosis of diabetic foot neuroarthropathy was based on the presence of distal sensory neuropathy, hyperglycemia, and characteristic radiographic and scintigraphic changes. The patient had only a partial response to a molded orthotic insert and medical management of the diabetes mellitus.

Clinical Pearls

1. Neuroarthropathy, or Charcot joint, may occur in association with a variety of central or peripheral nervous system diseases.

2. Tabes dorsalis, once the most frequent cause of neuroarthropathy, generally affects the knee, hip, ankle or spine.

3. Diabetes mellitus is now the most frequent underlying cause of neuroarthropathy, usually affecting the joints of the forefoot and midfoot.

4. Neuroarthropathy is occasionally the initial clinical manifestation of diabetes mellitus.

5. Consider the diagnosis in the patient with sensory neuropathy and radiographs showing osseous fragmentation, sclerosis, subluxation, or dislocation with joint disorganization.

REFERENCES

1. Resnick D. Neuroarthropathy, In: Resnick D, Niwayama G (eds). Diagnosis of Bone and Joint Disorders. Philadelphia, WB Saunders 1988, pp 3154–3187.
2. Papa J, Myerson M, Girard P. Salvage, with arthrodesis, in intractable diabetic neuropathic arthropathy of the foot and ankle. J Bone Joint Surg (Am) 1993; 75:1056–1066.
3. Pedersen LM, Madsen OR, Bliddal H. Charcot arthropathy as an unusual initial manifestation of diabetes mellitus. Br J Rheumatol 1993; 32:854–855.
4. Myerson MS, Henderson MR, Saxby T, Short KW. Management of midfoot diabetic neuroarthropathy. Foot Ankle Int 1994; 15:233–241.
5. Sequeira W. The neuropathic joint. Clin Exp Rheumatol 1994; 12:325–337.
6. Schauweeker DS. Differentiation of infected from noninfected rapidly progressive neuropathic osteoarthropathy. J Nucl Med 1995; 36:1427–1428.

PATIENT 62

A 10-year-old boy with a painful, swollen foot

A 10-year-old boy comes to the emergency department complaining of pain and swelling of 10-day duration in his right foot. About two weeks ago he sustained a puncture wound to this foot while wearing sneakers. Two days later he noted pain and swelling and was treated with cephalexin by his pediatrician. However, his symptoms persisted, and he is now unable to walk on the foot. The patient denies fever, chills, or malaise. Past medical history is unremarkable. He has no known allergies.

Physical Examination: Temperature 37°; pulse 90; respirations 12; blood pressure 110/60. General: no acute distress. HEENT: no abnormalities. Cardiac: regular rhythm, no murmur. Chest: clear. Abdomen: soft, nontender, positive bowel sounds. Extremities: plantar surface of right foot erythematous, tender, and swollen.

Laboratory Examination: Hct 36%; WBC 18,000/μl with 90% neutrophils, 5% bands, 5% lymphocytes; platelets 200,000/μl; ESR 70 mm/hr. Radiograph of foot: negative. Technetium bone scan: positive.

Question: What is your diagnosis?

Diagnosis: *Pseudomonas* osteochondritis

Discussion: *Pseudomonas aeruginosa* is the most common cause of osteochondritis involving the cartilage, small joints, and bones of the foot. *Pseudomonas* osteochondritis was first described after puncture wounds of the foot in children wearing sneakers, and *Pseudomonas* has been isolated from the soles of the sneakers. Patients usually present a week after the injury, and therapy with routine antibiotics used for cellulitis often has failed. There may be early improvement in pain and swelling after the puncture wound, followed by worsening symptoms several days later. The most common presentation is a swollen, tender foot. Examination of the plantar surface may reveal cellulitis and sometimes drainage. Patients usually are afebrile, and systemic symptoms typically are absent. Radiographs may be negative early on in the disease, but **bone scans** should be positive. The diagnosis is confirmed by growing *P. aeruginosa* from an aspiration of the affected area. Infection can involve the proximal phalanges/metatarsals, tarsal bones, and calcaneus.

Treatment consists of **surgical debridement** and **antipseudomonal antibiotics,** such as pipericillin or ceftazidime, combined with gentamicin. The length of therapy is controversial. Some patients respond to a short course (1–2 weeks); however, relapses can occur.

In the present patient, the radiograph of the foot was negative for osteomyelitis, but a bone scan was positive. Aspiration of the foot revealed a small amount of purulent material which grew *P. aeruginosa.* He was treated with a 3-week course of pipericillin and gentamicin plus surgical debridement, with a good response.

Clinical Pearls

1. Sneakers are the source of *Pseudomonas aeruginosa* in osteochondritis following puncture wounds.
2. Systemic symptoms such as fever and chills usually are absent.
3. Technetium scan almost always is positive in *Pseudomonas* osteochondritis, but radiographs can be negative.

REFERENCES

1. Jacobs RF, Adelman L, Sack CM, et al: Management of *Pseudomonas* osteochondritis complicating puncture wounds of the foot. Pediatrics 1982; 69:432–435.
2. Fisher MC, Goldsmith JF, Gilligan PH: Sneakers as a source of *Pseudomonas aeruginosa* in children with osteomyelitis following puncture wounds. J Pediatr 1985; 106:607–609.
3. Jacobs RF, McCarthy RE, Elsen JM: *Pseudomonas* osteochondritis complicating puncture wounds of the foot in children: A 10 year evaluation. J Infect Dis 1989; 160:657–661.

PATIENT 63

A 30-year-old man with painful, warm, spreading cellulitis of the leg

A 30-year-old man comes to the emergency department complaining of a painful right leg. Two days earlier he was bitten by an insect on his lower leg. The next day he noted redness and swelling around the bite, and these symptoms rapidly spread up his leg. His past medical history is unremarkable, and he has no known allergies.

Physical Examination: Temperature 39.4°; pulse 120; respirations 12; blood pressure 130/80. General: moderate distress. HEENT: no pharyngitis. Neck: supple. Cardiac: no murmur. Abdomen: soft, nontender, normal bowel sounds. Extremities: erythematous right leg, swollen and tender (see figure).

Laboratory Findings: Hct 36%; WBC 21,000/μl with granulocytes 80%, bands 10%; lymphocytes 10%; platelets 250,000/μl.

Question: What condition is suggested by the patient's clinical presentation?

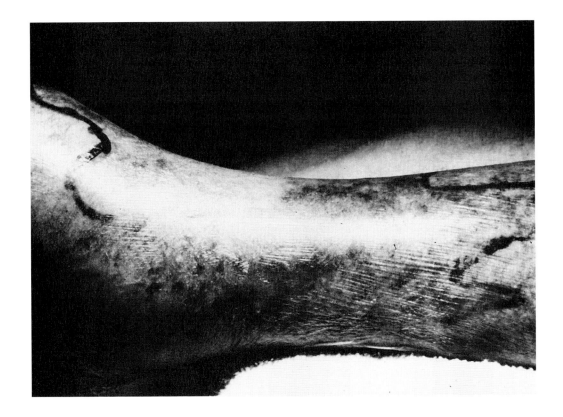

Diagnosis: Group A streptococcal cellulitis

Discussion: The group A streptococcus is a common cause of infections of the skin and soft tissues, especially impetigo, erysipelas, lymphangitis, and cellulitis. Streptococcal cellulitis is a **rapidly spreading inflammation** of the skin and subcutaneous tissues, usually occurring after trauma (sometimes mild or inapparent) or surgery. The patient develops fever, chills, malaise, local pain, erythema, and swelling, and there is a superficial desquamation of the skin overlying the area of cellulitis. Blood cultures may be positive for *S. pyogenes.*

Streptococcal cellulitis may be complicated by streptococcal toxic shock syndrome (TSS). Patients with streptococcal TSS most often have invasive soft tissue infections, rapidly developing hypotension, multiorgan failure, and sunburn-like macular rash. Most patients with streptococcal TSS are previously healthy individuals. Some cases have occurred in children due to secondary infection of varicella lesions with group A streptococcus.

Recurrent group A streptococcal cellulitis has occurred in patients with impaired lymphatic drainage. Women who have undergone a radical mastectomy are at risk for recurrent arm cellulitis. Recurrent leg cellulitis has developed in patients after coronary bypass surgery in the leg from which the saphenous vein was removed, especially in the presence of tinea pedis. Streptococci presumably gain entrance into the extremity through the small abrasions between the toes. Therapy involves treatment of the streptococcal infection as well as topical antifungal for the tinea pedis. Parenteral drug abusers also have an increased risk of streptococcal cellulitis, often associated with bacteremia, endocarditis, or septic thrombophlebitis.

Penicillin is the drug of choice for streptococcal cellulitis; however, cephalosporins providing broader coverage are a good choice for empiric therapy. In the penicillin-allergic patient, vancomycin or clindamycin are preferred.

The present patient was suspected to have streptococcal cellulitis of the leg on the basis of the bite history, rapid spread of erythema, and fever. Demonstration of *S. pyogenes* on blood culture confirmed the diagnosis. He was treated with cefazolin, 1 g intravenously every 8 hours, with prompt defervescence of his fever and rapid improvement of cellulitis over the next 7 days.

Clinical Pearls

1. Patients with impaired lymphatic drainage may have recurrent cellulitis.

2. Recurrent streptococcal leg cellulitis may occur in patients after coronary bypass surgery if the saphenous vein was removed.

3. Parenteral drug abusers have an increased risk of streptococcal cellulitis often associated with bacteremia, endocarditis, or septic thrombophlebitis.

REFERENCES

1. Stevens DL, Tanner MH, Winship J, et al: Severe group A streptococcal infections associated with a toxic shock-like syndrome and scarlet fever toxin. N Engl J Med 1989; 321:1–7.
2. Stevens DL: Invasive group A streptococcal infections. Clin Infect Dis 1991; 14:2–13.
3. Hoge CW, Schwartz B, Talkington DF, et al: The changing epidemiology of invasive group A streptococcal infections and the emergence of streptococcal toxic shock-like symptoms: A retrospective population-based study. JAMA 1993; 269:384–389.

PATIENT 64

A 50-year-old diabetic man with a foot ulcer

A 50-year-old man with a history of diabetes mellitus complains of a nonhealing ulcer on the plantar surface of his left foot. He first noted the ulcer about 2 weeks prior to his visit, after discovering a purulent discharge staining his sock. In addition, he has experienced some swelling and redness of the dorsum of his foot. A low-grade fever has been present for 2–3 days. He denies any pain, and cannot recall any specific trauma to the area. After noting the ulcer, he had visited a podiatrist who prescribed a "salve," but the patient did not keep his follow-up appointment. His past medical history is significant for diabetes mellitus of 15-year duration, with known complications of peripheral neuropathy, retinopathy, and chronic renal insufficiency. He is currently taking glyburide and captopril for hypertension. He denies any drug allergies.

Physical Examination: Temperature 37.8°; pulse 84; respirations 14; blood pressure 160/95. HEENT: extensive retinal scarring due to prior laser photocoagulation. Cardiac: normal. Abdomen: unremarkable. Extremities: hairless below knees, multiple ecchymoses in various stages of resolution, dorsalis pedis and posterior tibial pulses diminished bilaterally, 2+ right pedal edema with overlying erythema; well-circumscribed, punched-out ulcer approximately 2½ inches in diameter on plantar surface of left foot over area of second metatarsal head, with devitalized tissue and purulent discharge.

Laboratory Findings: WBC 15,300/µl with 88% neutrophils, 2% bands, 9% lymphocytes, 1% monocytes. BUN 24 mg/dl, creatinine 2.3 mg/dl. ESR 98 mm/hr. Culture of foot ulcer: *Staphylococcus aureus, S. epidermidis, Escherichia coli,* and *Enterococcus.* Radiograph of left foot: see figure.

Question: What is your diagnosis?

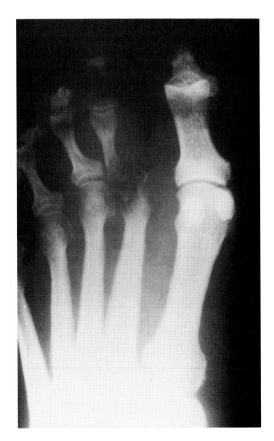

Diagnosis: Diabetic foot ulcer with chronic osteomyelitis

Discussion: Diabetic foot infections, when limited to the skin or superficial soft tissues, are caused by the same pathogens as in nondiabetics. These pathogens include *S. aureus,* streptococci, *E. coli* and other enteric gram-negative bacilli, and enterococci. In the diabetic patient with deep, penetrating infections, a variety of anaerobic pathogens such as *Peptostreptococcus, Peptococcus,* fusobacteria, and *Bacteroides* spp. must also be considered.

Diabetics presenting with deep, penetrating ulcers or chronic, draining sinus tracts of the foot almost always have an underlying chronic osteomyelitis. Even carefully taken cultures of the ulcer or sinus tract represent surface colonization and should not be equated with the underlying pathologic process or the presumed pathogenic organism. Only **bone biopsy cultures** are diagnostic and can be relied upon to select or change antibiotic therapy. Therefore, bone biopsy always should be performed. Prolonged empiric therapy should be avoided. **Extensive surgical debridement,** in addition to appropriate antimicrobial therapy, invariably is required for cure of chronic osteomyelitis. Inadequate debridement, in the hopes of preserving cosmesis, results in persistent or worsening infection despite prolonged antibiotics.

Initial empiric antibiotic therapy should consist of a broad-spectrum agent that has activity against the organisms mentioned above. Monotherapy with a third-generation cephalosporin (e.g., cefotaxime, ceftizoxime, cefoperazone) or a penicillin-β-lactamase inhibitor combination (e.g., ampicillin/sulbactam, piperacillin/tazobactam, ticarcillin/clavulanate) provides appropriate coverage. In the penicillin-allergic patient, clindamycin in combination with an aminoglycoside, quinolone, or aztreonam is recommended. Generally, monotherapy with an older quinolone should not be relied upon because of potential development of resistance, especially in staphylococci. Trovafloxacin, a broad-spectrum quinolone, is an exception to this rule. Although a small percentage of diabetic foot infections are caused by *Pseudomonas aeruginosa,* empiric coverage for this organism is not warranted. *P. aeruginosa* should be suspected, however, in cases following puncture wounds through a sneaker, and double *Pseudomonas* coverage should be initiated pending culture in this situation.

The present patient's foot ulcer—of prolonged duration—in combination with a **markedly elevated ESR** is suspicious for an underlying osteomyelitis. The destructive bony changes on radiograph confirm the diagnosis. If the radiograph had been nondiagnostic, a technetium bone scan would have been indicated. The patient underwent a ray amputation of the second phalanx and distal metatarsal bone. While an inpatient, he was given a week of IV ampicillin/sulbactam, which subsequently was changed to an oral combination of clindamycin and ofloxacin for an additional 3 weeks outpatient.

Clinical Pearls

1. In a diabetic with a nonhealing foot ulcer, an elevated ESR is suspicious for underlying osteomyelitis.

2. Superficial cultures rarely are helpful in establishing the pathogenic organism in osteomyelitis complicating a diabetic foot ulcer. A bone biopsy culture should be performed to direct antimicrobial therapy.

3. Extensive surgical debridement *always* is required for cure in cases of chronic osteomyelitis.

4. Empiric anti-*Pseudomonas* therapy is only necessary for patients who have experienced puncture wounds through a sneaker.

REFERENCES

1. Caputo GM, Cavanagh PR, Ulbrecht JS, et al: Diabetic foot infections. N Engl J Med 1994; 331:854–860.
2. Cunha BA: Diabetic foot infections. Infect Dis Pract 1994; 18:39.
3. Gibbens GW, Havershaw GM: Diabetic foot infections. Infect Dis Clin North Am 1995; 9:131–142.

PATIENT 65

A 55-year-old man with fever, erythema, and purulent drainage from the right leg

A 55-year-old man complains of fevers up to 38.3° C, worsening erythema, and purulent drainage from the lower medial aspect of his right leg. Symptoms commenced 4 days previously. His leg was injured at the same site in an automobile accident 5 years ago. He denies history of diabetes mellitus and is not taking any medication.

Physical Examination: Temperature 38°; pulse 86; respirations 16; blood pressure 142/82. General: well-developed, well-nourished man. Extremities: medial aspect of right lower leg swollen, erythematous, warm, and tender, with purulent drainage from a small opening. Chest: normal. Cardiac: unremarkable. HEENT: normal.

Laboratory Findings: WBC 14,800/μl with 83% polymorphonuclear cells, 16% lymphocytes, 1% monocytes; ESR 76 mm/hr. Gram stain of wound drainage: gram-positive cocci in clusters; identification pending. Blood cultures: negative. Computed tomography scan of right leg: see figure.

Question: What is your diagnosis?

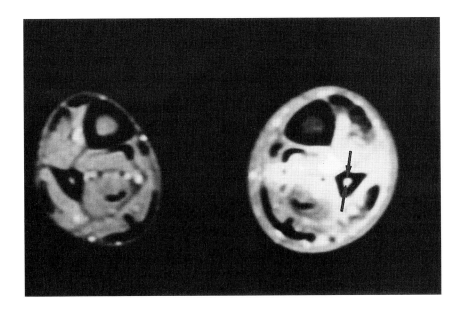

Diagnosis: Osteomyelitis due to *Staphylococcus aureus*

Discussion: Osteomyelitis is classified as acute or chronic depending on the clinical presentation and the radiologic and histologic findings. It also can be defined as hematogenous, secondary to a contiguous focus of infection, or associated with peripheral vascular insufficiency. Anatomically, osteomyelitis can be described as medullary, superficial, localized, or diffuse, depending on the extent of bony involvement. Acute hematogenous osteomyelitis is seen in children, but is uncommon in adults. It usually involves the vertebrae and rarely the long bones of the lower extremities. When the lower extremity is involved, affected areas are the metaphysis in children and the diaphysis in adults.

Immunocompromised persons and intravenous drug abusers are at highest risk for acquiring **acute hematogenous osteomyelitis** with bacteremic spread of infection, which can penetrate the cortical bone and lead to a soft tissue abscess. **Chronic hematogenous osteomyelitis** is more common than acute, and runs a protracted clinical course with recurrent reactivations of a quiescent focus and the eventual formation of sinus tracts. Osteomyelitis in adults typically is a result of a contiguous focus of infection secondary to trauma; nosocomial infection acquired during surgical procedures; insertion of a prosthesis; or spread from an overlying infected wound. By the time it presents, it usually is chronic. In an acute exacerbation of chronic osteomyelitis, patients present with fever, increased pain, swelling, and purulent drainage from an ulceration or sinus tract.

Patients may or may not have leukocytosis, but the erythrocyte sedimentation rate usually is elevated, and this finding can be used to monitor therapy. The purulent drainage should be cultured, and blood cultures should be drawn on all patients suspected of hematogenous osteomyelitis. The differential diagnosis of osteomyelitis includes malignant and benign tumors, past trauma, and bone infarcts from hemaglobulinopathies. Radiographs should be obtained in all patients suspected of osteomyelitis.

If the initial images are normal they should be repeated within 2 weeks, because the radiographic changes of osteomyelitis generally are delayed.

Typical findings in acute osteomyelitis include soft tissue swelling, periosteal thickening or elevation, and lytic changes. In chronic osteomyelitis, typical findings are sclerotic bone and periosteal reaction. Indium-labeled scans are useful for delineating the extent of bony destruction in acute osteomyelitis. However, magnetic resonance imaging (MRI) is the most sensitive test for chronic osteomyelitis. The pathogen most frequently isolated in hematogenous osteomyelitis is *Staphylococcus aureus*. Other organisms associated with the disorder include *S. epidermidis, Streptococcus pyogenes, Enterococcus* species, gram-negative bacilli, and anaerobes.

For chronic osteomyelitis, antibiotic treatment can be based on the results of bone, soft tissue, or blood cultures. Cultures should be obtained before antibiotic therapy is started or after the patient has been off antibiotics for 24–48 hours. In the treatment of chronic osteomyelitis, both antibiotics and surgical debridement are necessary for cure. At debridement, all necrotic bone and soft tissue should be removed, and antibiotic therapy should be based on the susceptibility of the organism isolated from bone cultures or deep bone biopsy. The patient should receive parenteral antibiotic therapy to complete a 4-week course after the last curative surgical debridement. Superficial osteomyelitis can be treated with a 2–4 week course of antibiotics after superficial debridement and flap surgery.

The present patient was admitted to the hospital and started on antibiotics for an acute exacerbation of cellulitis over chronically infected bone. Radiographs and MRI showed chronic osteomyelitis of the right tibia. Two weeks later, he underwent debridement of the involved bone, cultures of which grew *S. aureus*. The patient received a 6-week course of antibiotics.

Clinical Pearls

1. Acute hematogeneous osteomyelitis affecting the long bones is rare in adults.
2. In acute osteomyelitis, radiographic changes may be delayed and may actually show worsening although the patient is clinically improving.
3. The most common symptom of osteomyelitis is pain in the area of infection.
4. Acute osteomyelitis may be cured by antibiotics alone. Chronic osteomyelitis requires surgical debridement of infected bone for cure, and antibiotics are ancillary.

REFERENCES

1. Waldvogel FA, Medoff G, Swartz MN: Osteomyelitis: A review of clinical features, therapeutic considerations, and unusual aspects. N Engl J Med 1970; 282:198–206, 260–266, 316–322.
2. Waldvogel FA, Vasey H: Osteomyelitis: The past decade. N Engl J Med 1980; 303:360–370.
3. Mader JT, Calhoun J: Long bone osteomyelitis: Diagnosis and management. Hosp Practice 1994; 29:71–86.

PATIENT 66

A 33-year-old woman with a cold foot

A 33-year-old woman had a 1-day history of a cold right foot accompanied by pallor and paresthesias. She denied similar changes in the left foot or hands, although she had a 10-year history of episodic, triphasic color changes of the fingers and toes induced by cold exposure and complicated by digital ulcerations and calcinosis. She also had a long history of dysphagia and gastroesophageal reflux, "broken blood vessels" on the face, and hypertension. At the onset of the present illness she was taking nifedipine, enalapril, and omeprazole.

Physical Examination: Temperature 99.9°; heart rate 128; respiratory rate 18; blood pressure 100/60. Skin: telangiectasias over face and hands; sclerodactyly with healed digital pitted scars. HEENT: circumoral skin furrowing with decreased oral aperture. Chest: normal. Cardiac: normal. Neurologic: normal. Musculoskeletal: normal. Extremities: cold, pale right foot with no palpable pulse over the dorsalis pedis or posterior tibialis artery.

Laboratory Findings: WBC: 14,000/μL with 73% neutrophils, 17% lymphocytes, 10% monocytes. Hct 43.8%; platelets 362,000/μL; ESR 4 mm/hr. Serum chemistries: normal. Urinalysis: normal. Chest radiograph: normal. Echocardiogram: normal. Antiphospholipid antibody and lupus anticoagulant: negative. PT and PTT: normal. Cryoglobulins: negative. ANA: positive, 1:320 centromere pattern. Arteriogram: see below.

Question: What is the diagnosis and treatment?

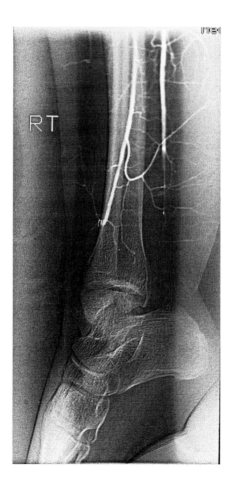

Diagnosis: CREST syndrome with large vessel occlusive disease.

Discussion: Systemic sclerosis (SSc, scleroderma) is classified by the extent of cutaneous involvement and the presence or absence of features of other connective tissue diseases, e.g., systemic lupus erythematosus, polymyositis, and dermatomyositis. In this classification, scleroderma exists as diffuse cutaneous SSc, limited cutaneous SSc, or an overlap syndrome. Patients with limited cutaneous SSc usually have taut skin on the fingers (sclerodactyly) and face and sometimes on the hand and forearm. Many patients with limited cutaneous SSc have Raynaud's phenomenon as the presenting symptom and develop calcinosis, esophageal dysmotility, sclerodactyly, and telangiectasia over the course of many years. This constellation of signs and symptoms is known by the acronym CREST. Approximately 50% of CREST syndrome patients have anticentromere antibodies (ACA).

Obliterative microvascular disease and vasospastic phenomena are hallmarks of SSc, but large vessel occlusive disease is reported infrequently. It would appear, however, that macrovascular disease is more prevalent among SSc patients than in control populations. Large vessel disease may present, as in the present case, with acute pallor and pain due to arterial occlusion, or as intermittent claudication, angina and transient ischemic attacks. Coexisting hypertension, diabetes or hypercholesterolemia may play a role in some cases. Antiphospholipid antibodies, or the lupus anticoagulant, may contribute to large and medium-sized vascular occlusion in some SSc patients. In other cases, such as the present patient, neither atherosclerosis nor antiphospholipid antibodies are detectable. Tests for the lupus anticoagulant and antiphospholipid antibodies were negative, and there was no arteriographic evidence of atherosclerosis. The arteriogram revealed normal vascular anatomy to the level of the right calf, at which point the anterior tibial artery was found to be occluded; the peritoneal and posterior tibial arteries were occluded at the level of the ankle, without arteriographic evidence of atherosclerosis or vasculitis (see figure).

Medical management of ischemic episodes is often difficult and ineffective. Digital ischemia may respond to vasodilator therapy including calcium-channel blockers, topical nitroglycerin, and chemical sympathectomy. Low-dose aspirin may inhibit platelet aggregation, and pentoxifylline may increase red blood cell flow. Surgical debridement or amputation is sometimes required.

Thrombolytic agents have been shown to improve symptoms and skin blood flow in SSc patients with digital ischemia, but there is little reported experience with thrombolytic therapy for large vessel occlusive disease in SSc patients. In the present case, a microcatheter was advanced into the posterior tibial artery to the level of the occlusion and a bolus of urokinase was given, followed by continuous infusion of urokinase and heparin. Within 24 hours, the foot was warm and the pulses were palpable. Repeat angiography demonstrated a patent posterior tibial artery and plantar arcades reconstituting the distal dorsalis pedis artery. The patient was placed on long-term coumadin therapy.

Clinical Pearls

1. Systemic sclerosis (SSc, scleroderma) is classified by the extent of skin involvement as limited cutaneous or diffuse cutaneous SSc or as an overlap variant with features of systemic lupus erythematosus or poly/dermatomyositis.

2. The limited cutaneous variant of SSc is also known as the CREST syndrome.

3. Approximately 50% of patients with limited cutaneous SSc have the specific anticentromere antibody.

4. Large vessel occlusive disease may occur in SSc patients, particularly those with the CREST variant.

5. Factors contributing to large vessel occlusive disease in some SSc patients include hypertension, atherosclerosis, and antiphospholipid antibodies.

6. Ischemia from large vessel occlusive disease can be improved by thrombolytic therapy.

REFERENCES

1. Shapiro LS. Large vessel arterial thrombosis in systemic sclerosis associated with antiphospholipid antibodies. J Rheumatol 1990; 17:685–688.

2. Klimuik PS, Kay EA, Illingworth KJ, Gush RJ, Taylor LJ, Baker RD, Perkins C, Jayson MIV. A double blind placebo controlled trial of recombinant tissue plasminogen activator in the treatment of digital ischemia in systemic sclerosis. J Rheumatol 1992; 19:716–720.

3. Youssef P, Englert H, Bertouch J. Large vessel occlusive disease associated with CREST syndrome and scleroderma. Ann Rheum Dis 1993; 52:464–466.

4. Veale DJ, Collidge TA, Belch JJF. Increased prevalence of symptomatic macrovascular disease in systemic sclerosis. Ann Rheum Dis 1995; 54:853–855.

PATIENT 67

A 50-year-old tennis player with acute calf pain

A 50-year-old man felt a sudden, painful tearing sensation in the calf during the first game of a tennis match. The pain was worse when the foot was plantarflexed, then suddenly dorsiflexed. There was immediate swelling of the calf, and he could not continue playing tennis. One day later the lower leg and foot appeared bruised. Pain and swelling persisted for weeks, and he sought medical attention.

Physical Examination: Vital signs: normal. General examination: normal. Extremities: full range of motion of knees and ankles; 2 cm asymmetry of calf circumference, right greater than left; tender to palpation at musculotendinous junction of right medial gastrocnemius muscle.

Laboratory Findings: CBC, coagulation tests, serum chemistries: normal. MRI of legs: see figure.

Question: What is the cause of this tennis player's leg pain?

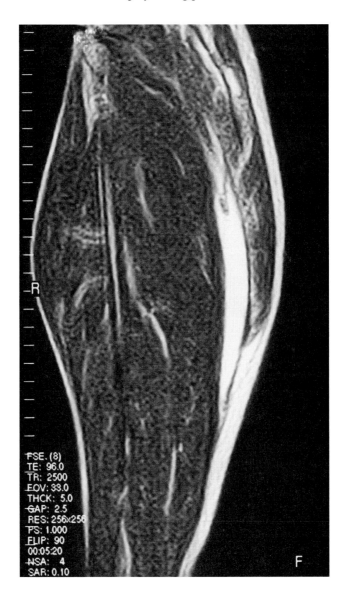

Diagnosis: Rupture of the plantaris muscle, or "tennis leg."

Discussion: Strains or tears of the plantaris muscle or of the medial head of the gastrocnemius muscle, sometimes referred to as "tennis leg," are seen in tennis players older than 40 years. Similar injuries in middle-aged persons engaged in other athletic endeavors, such as skiing or stair-stepping exercises have been observed. Typically, the individual experiences a sudden, painful tearing sensation in the calf muscle with immediate disability and swelling, followed by ecchymosis progressing down the leg into the ankle and foot. Palpation may reveal minimal swelling in a first-degree strain, ranging to a defect in the medial head of the gastrocnemius at the musculotendinous juncture in a severe strain. Conventional radiography and bone scanning have little value in the diagnosis of soft tissue injury. Ultrasonography and MRI scanning may demonstrate fluid collections and muscle tears. As shown in the Figure, an MRI scan reveals an intramuscular hematoma between the soleus muscle and the medial head of the gastrocnemius. The plantaris muscle, which is absent in 7 to 10% of the population, ranges from 7 to 13 cm long, with the myotendinous junction occurring at the level of the origin of the soleus muscle in the proximal portion of the lower leg.

Other causes of acute calf pain to be considered include dissection or rupture of a popliteal cyst; rupture of the Achilles tendon; and deep vein thrombosis. The latter is more likely to occur in a sedentary individual, whereas all of the former conditions typically occur during exercise. Rupture or dissection of a popliteal cyst is usually antedated by knee swelling. Rupture of the Achilles tendon usually occurs 1 to 2 inches proximal to the distal attachment of the tendon on the calcaneus. A characteristic "pop" sensation is felt, with an inability to stand on tiptoes. A positive Thompson test (failure of plantar flexion with passive compression of the gastrocnemius on the affected side) is present with rupture of the Achilles tendon but not with strain or tear of the medial head of the gastrocnemius.

Acute care of plantaris or gastrocnemius muscle strain consists of ice, restricted activity, gentle stretching exercises, heel lifts, and a progressive strengthening program. Immobilization and non-weight-bearing may be necessary in more severe cases to allow complete healing of the muscle.

In the present case, complete recovery occurred following a period of restricted activity.

Clinical Pearls

1. "Tennis leg" refers to strains or tears of the plantaris muscle or of the medial head of the gastrocnemius, usually occurring in tennis players over the age of 40, but also occurring in other athletic activities.

2. Consider the diagnosis in the athlete complaining of sudden, painful tearing sensation in the calf muscles with immediate swelling followed by ecchymosis progressing down the leg.

3. The differential diagnosis includes rupture of a popliteal cyst, rupture of the Achilles tendon, or deep vein thrombosis.

4. MR imaging may reveal an intermuscular hematoma between the soleus muscle and the medial head of the gastrocnemius muscle; an associated partial tear of the medial head of the gastrocnemius muscle also may be observed.

REFERENCES

1. Gilbert T, Ansari A. A tennis player with a swollen calf. Hosp Pract 1991;26:209–210,212.
2. Menz MJ, Lucas GL. Magnetic resonance imaging of a rupture of the medial head of the gastrocnemius muscle. A case report. J Bone Joint Surg (Am) 1991;73:1260–1262.
3. O'Neil R. Chapter 7. Foot, ankle and lower leg. In: Anderson MK, Hall SJ (eds). Sports Injury Management. Baltimore, Williams & Wilkins, 1995, pp 248–249.
4. Helms CA, Fritz RC, Garvin GJ. Plantaris muscle injury: evaluation with MR imaging. Radiology 1995;195:201–203.

PATIENT 68

A 54-year-old man with painful thigh muscles

A 54-year-old man with a 5-year history of diabetes mellitus and coronary artery disease developed bilateral thigh pain. Two weeks later the left anterior thigh became indurated and more painful. He had no weakness, but the severity of the pain limited walking. His only medication was glyburide.

Physical Examination: Vital signs: normal. Extremities: induration of the left lateral thigh with exquisite tenderness of both quadriceps muscles.

Laboratory Findings: WBC 13,500/μL with 60% neutrophils, 13% lymphocytes, 7% monocytes; Hct 40%; platelet count 303,000/μL. Electrolytes, BUN, creatinine, and liver function tests: normal. Urinalysis: 100 mg/dL protein, 500 mg/dL glucose. CPK: 109 IU/mL (44–180). Westergren ESR: 92 mm/hr. Biopsy of left lateral quadriceps femoris muscle (see figure).

Question: What is the diagnosis?

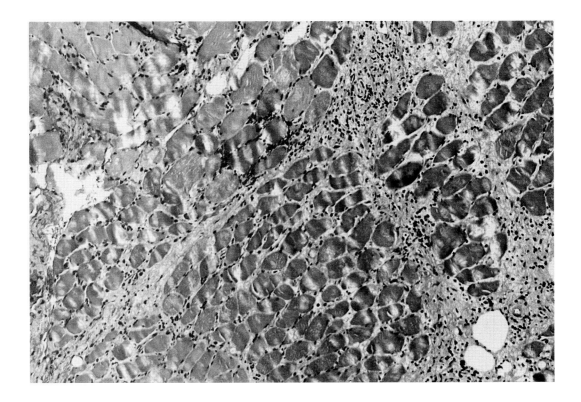

Diagnosis: Diabetic muscle infarction.

Discussion: Subacute, painful, and swollen muscle can result from only a few pathologic processes. Intramuscular hemorrhage from trauma or a coagulation defect can cause this picture, but is easily excluded by history and laboratory testing. Tropical pyomyositis resulting from staphylococcal infection is seen only in the tropics and is the result of spread from a localized skin infection. Inflammatory muscle disease (poly- or dermatomyositis) is characterized by weakness rather than pain, and is associated with proximal more than distal musculature. One unusual form of inflammatory muscle disease is "localized myositis" in which just one muscle or muscle group is involved. The pathologic features are those of idiopathic inflammatory muscle disease: inflammatory cell infiltrate with degeneration and regeneration of muscle fibers. Diabetic muscle infarction is the other entity to be considered in this setting.

Diabetic muscle infarction generally occurs in patients with longstanding, poorly controlled diabetes mellitus. The clinical picture is that of a painful, swollen, and tender thigh, either unilateral or bilateral. Most patients are insulin-dependent, and the first patients to be described had evidence of end-organ involvement, particularly renal disease with proteinuria or uremia. More recent case reports include type II diabetics, but most have atherosclerosis and poor glycemic control. The pathologic findings on biopsy are muscle necrosis and inflammation (see figure).

Treatment of diabetic muscle infarction includes analgesics and glycemic control, with rehabilitation when pain subsides. Immunosuppression is not beneficial, and corticosteroids may only worsen the situation.

The present patient had been started on steroids initially, as he was believed to have had localized myositis. There was no improvement over a 6-week period, and control of his glucose became quite difficult. Prednisone was stopped, pain control was instituted, and gentle physical therapy was begun. He improved gradually over a 4-month period.

Clinical Pearls

1. Diabetic muscle infarction occurs in the setting of poorly controlled diabetes, most often in patients with evidence of end-organ damage.

2. Patients with diabetic muscle infarction complain of severe unilateral or bilateral thigh pain. Swelling, induration, and erythema of the quadriceps muscle are characteristic.

3. Treatment of diabetic muscle infarction involves analgesics, control of blood glucose, and gentle exercise. Corticosteroids are not helpful and should be avoided.

REFERENCES

1. Barton KL, Palmer BF. Bilateral infarction of the vastus lateralis muscle in a diabetic patient: a case report and review of the literature. J Diabetes Complications 1993;7:221–223.
2. Rocca PV, Alloway JA, Nashel DJ. Diabetic muscular infarction. Semin Arthritis Rheum 1993;22:280–287.
3. Bodner RA, Younger DS, Rosoklija G. Diabetic muscle infarction. Muscle Nerve 1994;17:949–950.
4. Bjornskov EK, Carry MR, Katz FH, et al. Diabetic muscle infarction: a new perspective on pathogenesis and management. Neuromuscul Disord 1995;5:39–45.

PATIENT 69

A 33-year-old woman with heel pain

A 33-year-old woman with a 1-year history of right heel pain was seen. She denied traumatic injury, but stated she worked in a textile mill on her feet for up to 14 hours daily. She had no other musculoskeletal complaints. She denied having a rash, eye inflammation, or dysuria. The patient remembered having a 3-week diarrheal illness before onset of the heel pain and still notes loose stools twice weekly. Her father had an inflammatory arthritis of the right elbow.

Physical Examination: Vital signs: normal. Skin: normal. HEENT: normal. Cardiopulmonary: normal. Abdomen: normal. Neurologic: normal. Musculoskeletal: thickened, tender right Achilles tendon with atrophy of the calf, pain on dorsiflexion and inversion of the right foot, and painful plantar fascia. Schöber index: normal.

Laboratory Findings: CBC: normal. Uric acid: normal. RF: negative. ANA: negative. Westergren ESR: 6 mm/hr. HLA B-27: positive. HIV: negative. Sacroiliac radiographs: normal. Ankle radiographs: small plantar spur and slight opacification of the pre-Achilles fat triangle suggestive of inflammation. MRI (shown below): increased signal intensity within the distal right Achilles tendon measuring 1.3 cm in transverse diameter.

Question: What is the cause and treatment of this patient's heel pain?

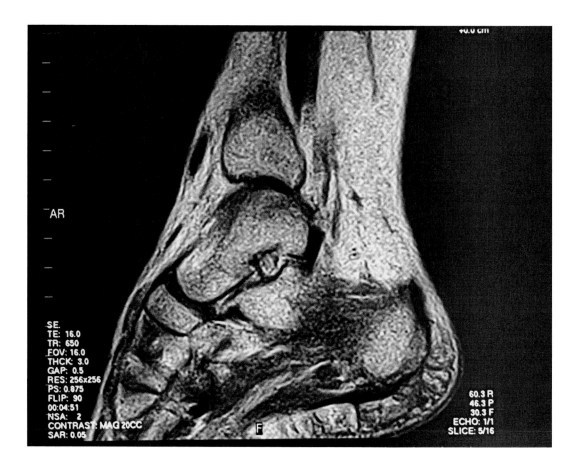

Diagnosis: Incomplete Reiter's syndrome.

Discussion: Reiter's syndrome classically refers to peripheral arthritis, nonspecific urethritis and conjunctivitis following a dysenteric illness or venereal disease. Reiter's syndrome is a reactive arthritis that occurs in a genetically susceptible host (HLA-B27 positive) following infection of the gut by Salmonella, Shigella, Yersinia, or Campylobacter, or of the genitourinary tract by Chlamydia. An incomplete form of Reiter's syndrome occurs as an asymmetric oligoarthritis of the lower extremities without urethritis or conjunctivitis.

One should consider the diagnosis of Reiter's syndrome in any patient with an asymmetric oligoarthritis involving lower extremity joints, especially if there is heel pain. Unlike rheumatoid arthritis, Reiter's syndrome is asymmetric and has a predilection for lower extremity joints. Patients with Reiter's syndrome are RF negative, and the ESR is often normal.

Occasional patients with long-standing Reiter's syndrome develop axial disease and, like patients with ankylosing spondylitis, have limited lumbar flexion and abnormal Schöber test. The Schöber test entails a measurement of 10 cm over the lumbar area with the patient erect. An increase of less than 5 cm when the patient is asked to touch the floor implies inability to reverse the lumbar lordosis and is often seen in patients with seronegative spondyloarthropathy.

Another feature of seronegative spondyloarthropathy, including Reiter's syndrome, is its tendency to cause inflammation at tendinous insertions into bone; this is called **enthesopathy.** This gives rise to the "sausage digit" in the hands or feet, as well as to Achilles tendinitis and plantar fasciitis in the foot. Similar findings may be seen in the other HLA-B27 related conditions: ankylosing spondylitis, psoriatic arthritis, and inflammatory bowel disease.

Achilles tendinitis due to Reiter's syndrome gives rise to chronic hind foot swelling and pain (talalgia). Other causes of acute or chronic Achilles tendinitis include trauma, athletic overuse, RA, gout, pseudogout, xanthomas in hyperlipoproteinemias, and the other HLA-B27 associated conditions. The presence of heel pain often correlates with a poor prognosis and may lead to work disability.

Plain radiographs, ultrasound, and MRI may be useful to demonstrate Achilles tendinitis. In normal individuals the thickness of the Achilles tendon is between 4 and 8 mm at the level of the calcaneus. With inflammation, the tendon is thickened. An associated retrocalcaneal bursitis may obliterate the normal radiolucency that extends at least 2 mm below the posterosuperior surface of the calcaneus.

Treatment of Achilles tendinitis includes NSAIDs, heel support, splinting (ankle-foot orthosis), and gentle stretching. The Achilles tendon is vulnerable to rupture and must not be injected with corticosteroid, but retrocalcaneal bursitis and plantar fasciitis may respond to injected corticosteroid. Resistant cases may improve with sulfasalazine, methotrexate, or azathioprine. Reiter's disease may be the presenting manifestation of human immunodeficiency virus (HIV) infection. In such cases, it is usually incomplete with enthesopathy and fasciitis of the feet being dominant features. Immunosuppressive therapy is contraindicated in HIV-positive patients. Local radiotherapy to the heel may yield prompt and persistent improvement in cases refractory to conservative treatment.

In the present case, a diagnosis of incomplete Reiter's syndrome was made in this young woman who was HLA-B27 positive with Achilles tendinitis following a diarrheal illness. Ileocolonoscopy was negative for inflammatory bowel disease. Achilles tendinitis failed to respond to NSAIDs, orthotics, sulfasalazine, and methotrexate. Soft tissue swelling resolved with local radiotherapy, but pain and disability persisted.

Clinical Pearls

1. Talalgia, or heel pain, may be the first symptom of seronegative spondyloarthropathy: Reiter's syndrome, ankylosing spondylitis, psoriatic arthritis, inflammatory bowel disease.

2. Reiter's syndrome (arthritis, nonspecific urethritis, and conjunctivitis) may present with arthritis alone (incomplete Reiter's syndrome), in which case heel pain is usually a prominent feature.

3. Incomplete Reiter's syndrome, especially enthesopathy and fasciitis of the feet, may be a manifestation of human immunodeficiency virus (HIV) infection.

4. Heel pain secondary to Reiter's syndrome is often chronic and may be disabling.

5. Radiographic features of Reiter's syndrome involving the heel include thickening of the Achilles tendon, obliteration of the retrocalcaneal recess, ill-defined spurs, and/or erosions of the plantar and posterior aspects of the calcaneus.

6. Refractory cases of Achilles tendinitis may respond to a course of local radiotherapy.

REFERENCES

1. Smith DL, Bennett RM, Regan MG. Reiter's disease in women. Arthritis Rheum 1980;23:335–340.
2. Gerster JC, Sandan Y, Fallet GH. Talalgia. A review of 30 severe cases. J Rheumatol 1978;5:210–216.
3. Resnick D, Feingold ML, Curd J, Ninayama G, Goergen TG. Calcaneal abnormalities in articular disorders. Radiology 1977;125:355–366.
4. Fox R, Calin A, Gerber RC, Gibson D. The chronicity of symptoms and disability in Reiter's syndrome. An analysis of 131 consecutive patients. Ann Intern Med 1979;91:190–193.
5. Winchester R. AIDS and the rheumatic diseases. Bull Rheum Dis 1990;39(5):1–10.
6. Grill V, Smith M, Ahern M, Littlejohn G. Local radiotherapy for pedal manifestations of HLA- B27-related arthropathy. Br J Rheumatol 1988;27:390–392.

PATIENT 70

A 40-year-old diabetic man with a persistent ulcer

A 40-year-old man with chronic diabetes mellitus is referred for an evaluation of a chronic ulceration on his left foot. The ulcer has been present for 8 months, with a gradual increase in length, width, and depth. The increase in size has continued despite weekly debridements. Past medical history includes a right leg below-the-knee amputation, due to an "uncontrolled infection."

Physical Examination: Vascular (left lower extremity): intact tree. Palpation: dorsalis pedis and posterior tibial pulses evident. Skin: 6 cm × 5 cm × 7 cm plantar ulceration located beneath cuboid bone; superficial, no clinical signs of infection.

Laboratory Findings: Tc-99 bone scan: negative for osteomyelitis. Radiographs: significant amount of joint subluxation and shifting; especially in mid-foot region. Blood work (including CBC with differential): normal.

Questions: What is the likely cause of an ulceration of this size in this location? What is the explanation for the delayed healing—especially in the presence of intact circulation?

Diagnosis: Charcot diabetic osteoarthropathy

Discussion: A chronic, non-healing ulcer in this location is very common, especially in the presence of a collapsed mid-foot. The absence of the contralateral limb accentuates the weight-bearing pressures and the vertical forces on the remaining foot. As a result, especially in the presence of sensory neuropathy, the lack of the "protective feedback mechanism" may be devastating.

The accepted treatment for acute neuropathic arthropathy of the foot and/or ankle in patients with diabetes has been prolonged immobilization in a brace or plaster cast until consolidation and healing are evident radiographically, and clinical stability of the foot and ankle has been restored. This method is effective in most patients, especially when treatment is instituted early, before a fixed deformity has developed. However, despite prompt immobilization and protected weight bearing, severe deformities develop in some patients. Also, after some neuropathic dislocations of the peritalar or ankle joint, whether acute or chronic, the feet are too unstable to be maintained in adequate alignment by either a brace or a plaster cast. In addition, some patients may not seek treatment until after disabling, fixed deformities have developed. Deformed neuropathic extremities, if subjected to the stresses of weight bearing, are susceptible to ulceration and infection as well as to the risk of eventual amputation.

Operative treatment is occasionally warranted to avoid these sequelae. Enthusiasm for operative treatment has generally been tempered by the anticipated high frequency of pseudoarthroses and other complications. Numerous physicians have reported the results of operative treatment of neuropathic arthropathy, but most of these reports have concerned a single patient or a relatively small series. Nevertheless, useful information has been provided.

Shibata et al. reported the results of tibiotalar and tibiocalcaneal arthrodeses in 26 patients who had leprotic neuropathic arthropathy. With an intramedullary nail used for fixation, fusion was successful in 19 patients. The complications included seven pseudoarthroses and four infections, and two patients eventually had an amputation.

Stuart and Morrey reported the results of arthrodesis of the ankle and peritalar joints in 13 patients who had insulin-dependent diabetes mellitus, nine of whom had radiographic evidence of neuropathic arthropathy. The results were satisfactory in only five of the 13 patients, and there were complications in seven of the nine patients who had neuropathic changes. The complications included two nonunions and three deep infections, and there were also two below-the-knee amputations. However, a variety of operative techniques was employed for the arthrodeses in their series, and external fixation was used in nine of the 13 patients.

In summary, most patients who have neuropathic arthropathy can be managed satisfactorily with immobilization in a plaster cast or by an orthosis. Operative treatment is technically demanding and associated with a high rate of complications. However, when there is severe instability or a fixed deformity, open reduction and attempted arthrodesis with rigid fixation (see figures) may be the best way to salvage the extremity.

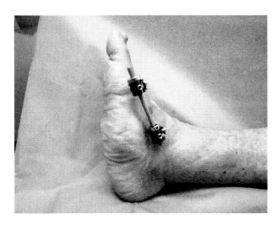 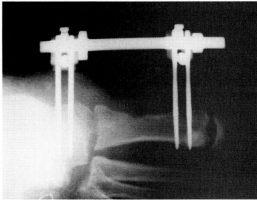

Clinical Pearls

1. Pursue any and all diagnostic studies to rule out infection in a patient with Charcot diabetic osteoarthropathy.

2. Determine the point of maximum weight-bearing pressure, and initiate a plan to "off-load" the pressure.

3. Devise a plan to trigger wound healing.

4. First attempt to off-load and possibly use an aperture-type cast, allowing weight bearing but without pressure on the deformity underlying the wound.

REFERENCES

1. Shibata T, Tada K, Hashizume C: The results of arthrodesis of the ankle for leprotic neuroarthropathy. J Bone Joint Surg 72-A: 749–756, 1990.
2. Stuart MJ, Morrey BF: Arthrodesis of the diabetic neuropathic ankle joint. Clin Orthop 253: 209–211, 1990.

INDEX